Systemic Sclerosis - Recent Advances and New Perspectives

Edited by Katja Lakota,
Katja Perdan Pirkmajer and Blaž Burja

Published in London, United Kingdom

Systemic Sclerosis - Recent Advances and New Perspectives
http://dx.doi.org/10.5772/intechopen.102205
Edited by Katja Lakota, Katja Perdan Pirkmajer and Blaž Burja

Contributors
Anja Srpčič, Bartosz Miziołek, Beata Bergler-Czop, Daniel E. Furst, Dwitya Elvira, Erin Chew, Felicita Urzi, Ganiat Adeogun, Katja Lakota, Katja Perdan Pirkmajer, Madeleine E. Frech, Mariela Geneva-Popova, Michał Szczepanek, Neža Brezovec, Preston M. McCourt, Rafael Contreras-Galindo, Raveinal Masri, S. Bobo Tanner, Sana Anwar, Sanie Dzambasova, Sanja Markez, Sergej Pirkmajer, Silvia Bellando-Randone, Souren Paul, Stanislava Popova-Belova, Tracy M. Frech, Velichka Popova, Vladimir Hodhzev, Yossra Suliman

First published in London, United Kingdom, 2024 by IntechOpen
IntechOpen is the global imprint of INTECHOPEN LIMITED, registered in England and Wales, registration number: 11086078, 5 Princes Gate Court, London, SW7 2QJ, United Kingdom

British Library Cataloguing-in-Publication Data
A catalogue record for this book is available from the British Library

Additional hard and PDF copies can be obtained from orders@intechopen.com

Systemic Sclerosis - Recent Advances and New Perspectives
Edited by Katja Lakota, Katja Perdan Pirkmajer and Blaž Burja
p. cm.
Print ISBN 978-1-83769-670-3
Online ISBN 978-1-83769-669-7
eBook (PDF) ISBN 978-1-83769-671-0

For EU product safety concerns:
IN TECH d.o.o., Prolaz Marije Krucifikse Kozulić 3, 51000 Rijeka, Croatia,
info@intechopen.com or visit our website at intechopen.com.

Meet the editors

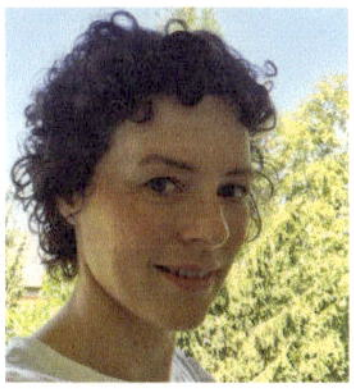

Katja Lakota, MPharm, Ph.D., received her Ph.D. in Biomedicine from the Faculty of Pharmacy, University of Ljubljana, Slovenia, in 2014 . She is a head of the national research program, Systemic Autoimmune Diseases, at the Department of Rheumatology, University Medical Centre Ljubljana, Slovenia. As Fulbright scholar, Dr. Lakota spent a research year in the laboratory of Prof. John Varga, Northwestern University, Chicago, USA, studying the role of adiponectin anti-fibrotic signaling in fibroblasts. She also investigated mechanisms leading to fibrosis development in systemic sclerosis during a post-doctoral fellowship from the Slovenian Research Agency in 2018. Dr. Lakota is an assistant professor in the Faculty of Mathematics, Natural Sciences and Information Technologies, University of Primorska, Slovenia, where she teaches courses on systems biology in human diseases.

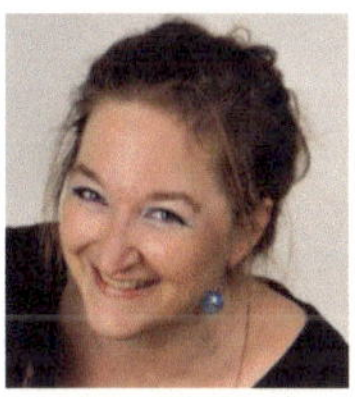

Katja Perdan Pirkmajer, MD, Ph.D., is a rheumatologist and clinical pharmacologist in the Rheumatology Department, University Medical Centre Ljubljana, Slovenia. She received her Ph.D. from the Faculty of Medicine, University of Ljubljana, Slovenia, in 2013. In addition to being a clinician and clinical researcher, she is also Assistant Professor of Internal Medicine at the Faculty of Medicine, University of Ljubljana. As a member of the Slovenian National Research Program in Systemic Autoimmune Diseases, she has conducted research on autoimmune responses after influenza vaccination, the predictive value of antiphospholipid antibodies, and the mechanisms of methotrexate action through 5-aminoimidazole-4-carboxamide ribonucleotide (AICAR) in patients with rheumatoid arthritis or psoriatic arthritis. Her current clinical and research work is now focused on systemic sclerosis in Sjögren's disease.

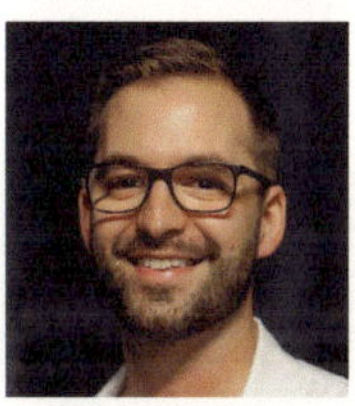

Blaž Burja, MD, Ph.D., is a physician-scientist at the Centre of Experimental Rheumatology, Department of Rheumatology, University Hospital Zurich, Switzerland, and an internal medicine resident at Cantonal Hospital Glarus, Switzerland. His research work focuses on translational science in systemic sclerosis, specifically on metabolic dysregulation in fibrosis and the development of novel anti-fibrotic therapies for fibrotic diseases. By performing basic science and translational research, Dr. Burja aims to bridge the bench-to-bedside gap and help to better understand and treat patients with fibrotic diseases.

Contents

Preface

Systemic sclerosis (SSc) is a rare autoimmune disease with one of the greatest impacts on patients' quality of life; patients with SSc have the highest morbidity and mortality among patients with rheumatic diseases. Therefore, intensive research is pursued to achieve better understanding of the pathophysiology of SSc, to find prognostic biomarkers and novel therapeutic strategies to improve patients' health and quality of living. This book describes the state of the art in the understanding of pathophysiology, diagnosis, and specific management of SSc clinical manifestations.

Chapter 1, "Current Update on the Role of Inflammation in the Pathogenesis of SSc", focuses on inflammatory activation in SSc and emphasizes the importance of oxidative stress in the initiation and progression of vasculopathy and fibrosis. Marked activation of the innate and adaptive immune system and an aberrant local immune response with autoimmune activation are considered as key profibrotic stimuli leading to the pathology of SSc.

Chapter 2, "Chromosome Segregation Defects in Scleroderma", describes the contribution of centromere and telomere dysfunction in SSc to chromosomal instability and the consequent activation of the cGAS/STING signaling pathway, leading to an inflammatory response. The preclinical symptoms, clinical presentation, and course of the disease are highly variable in SSc patients, and the characteristic skin thickening, allowing for definite diagnosis of SSc, sometimes appears very late. Early diagnosis of SSc can open a "window of opportunity" in management of the disease, but overtreatment of those who will not advance from initial symptoms should be avoided. Therefore, very early diagnosis of systemic sclerosis (VEDOSS) has been defined for individuals with Raynaud's phenomenon, autoantibodies, and SSc capillaroscopy pattern, who are likely to progress to definite SSc.

Chapter 3, "What Comes before Scleroderma?", emphasizes the need for further longitudinal studies to determine genetic and environmental risk factors and biomarkers for SSc patients to enable risk stratification and determine the benefit of early, preventive treatments.

Chapter 4, "Diagnostic Methods for Microvasculopathy in Systemic Sclerosis", focuses on microvasculopathy, which, in the form of Raynaud phenomenon, is usually the first clinical symptom of SSc. This chapter presents and discusses various methods for assessing microcirculation, including nailfold capilaroscopy, dermoscopy, laser Doppler method, and thermography.

Pulmonary involvement is common in SSc and is the major cause of death. Methods of SSc pulmonary involvement diagnosis and follow-up are always a matter of international discussions. Chapter 5, "Assessment of Lung Involvement and Prognostic Value of the 6-Minute Walking Test for Pulmonary Involvement in Patients with Systemic Sclerosis", describes serum biomarkers, imaging, and functional methods.

Furthermore, the chapter offers detailed description of the six-minute walk test, how to perform it, and how to interpret the results in SSc patients.

Chapter 6, "Important Considerations for Bone Health Management in Systemic Sclerosis Patients", explains why bone density is decreased in SSc patients, how bone health should be monitored, and what prevention and treatment options should be considered for SSc disease manifestations.

Skeletal muscle is affected in almost all SSc patients, but the presentation varies from myalgias and muscle weakness to fibrosing myopathy. In addition, myopenia/ sarcopenia occurs due to disease pathology, difficulty with physical exercise, and treatments. Chapter 7, "Skeletal Muscle Involvement in Systemic Sclerosis", describes all aspects of muscle involvement, including myokines.

Katja Lakota
Department of Rheumatology,
UMC Ljubljana,
Ljubljana, Slovenia

Katja Perdan Pirkmajer
Department of Rheumatology,
UMC Ljubljana,
Ljubljana, Slovenia

Faculty of Medicine,
University of Ljubljana,
Ljubljana, Slovenia

Blaž Burja
Department of Rheumatology,
University Hospital Zurich,
Switzerland

Chapter 1

Current Update on the Role of Inflammation in the Pathogenesis of SSc

Dwitya Elvira and Raveinal Masri

Abstract

Systemic sclerosis (SSc), also known as scleroderma, is a systemic autoimmune rheumatic disease characterized by dysregulation of the immune system, fibrosis of the skin and visceral organs, and vasculopathy. Inflammatory activation may be important in the initiation and progression of vasculopathy and fibrosis in response to homeostatic disturbance. Numerous factors trigger and enable sustained inflammation such as increased oxidative stress, involved in progressivity and disease severity. This chapter will focus on the role of inflammation and the involvement of multiple immune mediators contributing to autoimmune activity of SSc.

Keywords: autoimmune, inflammation, pathogenesis, scleroderma, systemic sclerosis

1. Introduction

Systemic sclerosis or scleroderma (SSc) is a systemic autoimmune disease characterized by a pathogenic triad: microangiopathy, immune dysfunction and fibrosis of the skin and visceral organs, in which chronic inflammation plays a crucial role and leads to the severity of organic lesions [1, 2]. The degree of skin fibrosis, immunological profile, and microvascular dysfunction determine the clinical classification of the disease, consisting of limited cutaneous SSc (lSSc) and diffuse cutaneous SSc (dSSc) disease subtype. dSSc is a devastating and serious disease with significant morbidity and mortality [2]. Scleroderma is now conceived as a complex disease with multiple pathogenic pathways. In particular, the central role of immune system cells and inflammatory mediators, fibroblasts and other cells determining the regulation of the extracellular matrix (ECM) is now recognized [3–5].

Dysregulations of the immune system were one of the first mechanisms recognized to be responsible for the onset of SSc [3]. An inflammatory process characterized by immune cell infiltration may be crucial in the initiation and progression of vasculopathy and fibrosis in response to homeostatic disturbance. The oxidative stress also increases the susceptibility of the disease [4–6]. One quarter of patient present with inflammatory signature, characterized by increased C-reactive protein and ESR, especially in early inflammatory phase of the disease. These biomarkers correlated with disease activity, severity, poor pulmonary function, and shorter survival [7]. Despite the increased acute-phase reactants that does not alter in treated patients, the inflammatory reactions in SSc are not as "highly inflammatory" as other rheumatic autoimmune diseases such as rheumatoid arthritis (RA) or systemic lupus erythematosus (SLE), whereas SSc usually shows less classical inflammatory signs such as rubor, calor, or dolor. Mitev et al. studied differences between patients with inflammatory SSc and non-inflammatory SSc, characterized by continuously elevated inflammatory biomarkers (ESR and CRP). Higher risk for SSc with high inflammatory biomarkers is present in older males, higher modified Rodnan skin score (mRSS), lower lung function compared to non-inflammatory SSc. Based on their study, macrophages of SSc with higher inflammatory markers were shown less affected with immunosuppressant treatment, thus maintaining the inflammation activity in inflammatory SSc patients [7, 8].

2. Innate immune system

A recent study demonstrated that Toll-like receptors (TLRs) are involved in SSc pathogenesis through two main mechanisms. The first mechanism is through increased of TLR expression due to persistent damage after viral infection with stimulation of interferon (IFN), transforming growth factors-β (TGF-β) and other mediators. The second mechanism is through the increased presence of damage-associated molecular patterns TLR agonists such as tenascin-C (TEN-C) and Fibronectin-EDA (FN-EDA) [9–14].

Persistent damage after viral infection could increase chronic inflammation by activation of dendritic cells by TLRs which leads to the production of several pro-inflammatory cytokines, [2] particularly type I interferon (IFN) which have been shown to be overexpressed in peripheral blood in patients with systemic sclerosis. Viral infection such as Epstein Barr-viruses activate TLR activation as an antiviral response against γ-herpes virus, which induces type I IFN and cytokines response. Interferons are multifunctional cytokines responsible for inducing cellular resistance to viruses. There is evidence of a strong IFN signature in SSc where nearly 50% of patients with SSc show the so-called "interferon signature (IFN signature)" in peripheral blood and sera [6]. It appears that the IFN signature in SSc may observed in the early phase of the disease, even before the skin fibrosis is well established. In early SSc, type I IFNs were thought to be responsible for the inflammatory process and activated mediators of fibrosis such as B-cell activating factor (BAFF) expression and serum levels of propeptide N-terminal type III procollagen. Increased expression of this type I IFN affects the function of immune and endothelial cells such as monocytes, as well as increased differentiation, survival, proliferation, and activation of T, B, dendritic cells, and fibroblasts. Increased expression of MxA (marker of IFN type I activity) and interferon regulatory factors (IRFs) also occurs in endothelial cells of SSc patients, correlated with the presence of ischemic ulcers digital [2, 6, 9–12].

The second mechanism on how TLR signaling may also be implicated in SSc pathogenesis is the presence of several agonists of TLR that are expressed in damaged cells of affected tissues and released into extracellular space. Tenascin-C (TEN-C) and Fibronectin-EDA (FN-EDA) were two of TLRs agonist identified as endogenous danger signal that drives TLRs signaling into upregulation of inflammation and fibrosis amplification in SSc. Tenascin-C is a multifactorial hexameric extracellular (ECM) glycoprotein consisting of 4 domains: a tenascin assembly (TA) domain, epidermal growth factor-like (EFGL) repeats, up to 17 FNIII-like repeats and a fibrinogen-like globe (FBG). Fibronectin-EDA (FN-EDA/fibronectin containing extra domain A) is cellular fibronectin expressed in endothelial cells that is associated with tissue remodeling, fibroblast differentiation, angiogenesis, and inflammation. Tenascin-C as a modulator of inflammatory response will stimulate the pro-inflammatory cytokine such as IL-6, IL-8, and TNF, meanwhile FN-EDA induced expression of multitude dermal fibroblast cytokines release from mast cells, such as CXCL-13, IL-8 and TNF-α. Tenascin-C and FN-EDA activate TLR4 activity in innate immune response, via TGF-B2 signaling lead to increase of fibrosis occurred in SSc [13–18].

3. The transition from innate immunity to adaptive immunity

Innate lymphoid cells (ILCs) are recently discovered innate immune cells that serve as first-line defense resembling the Th1, Th2, and Th17 in adaptive immunity. There are three types of ILC that have been described so far: ILC1, ILC2 and ILC3. These ILCs express MHC class II and possess transcription factors and cytokine profiles reminiscent of Th cells; ILC1 produces IFNγ; ILC2 produces IL-5, IL-9 and IL-13; ILC3 produces IL-17A and IL-22 [5, 6]. These cells act as antigen presenting cells (APC) like dendritic cells [6]. The role of ILCs as transition factors between innate and adaptive immunity in the pathogenesis of SSc is still an interesting topic of research. Dendritic cells also play a key role in the transition from innate to adaptive immunity through their ability to identify antigens from pathogen- or damage-associated molecular models (PAMPS or DAMPS) using TLRs, NLRs, RIG-I-like receptors (RLRs), and receptors for advanced glycation end products (RAGEs), thus process this information to T cells via the MHC-II/binding receptor complex antigen [6, 19, 20].

In SSc patients, ILC2 interaction with TGF-β could trigger profibrotic mechanisms of cutaneous fibroblast through increased of TGF-β and downregulation of Killer Cell Lectin-Like Receptor G (KLRG1). Binding of KLRG1 and ILC2 in circulation could migrate to the skin and pass to pro-fibrotic form, KLRG1 - ILC2, causing imbalance of anti-fibrotic and pro-fibrotic mediators and activate fibrosis mechanisms in skin fibroblast. ILC-2 produces IL-9 that shown to be increased in SSc patients, along with the increased of Th-9 lymphocytes, through mast cell-Th9-ILC2s. Activation of ILC-2 in stimulating chronic inflammation involves the secretion of alarmins, such as IL-33 cytokines, which play a central role in the modulation of ILC-2 and fibrosis in response to the initial inflammation phase in SSc [6, 19, 20].

4. Adaptive immunity

Several observations over several decades strongly imply a major role of the adaptive immune system in the pathogenesis of SSc. T cells are also present in the inflammatory tissue infiltrates of SSc patients which involve Th-1, Th-17 followed by a witch to Th-2 leading to irreversible fibrosis and 'burn-out' of disease. In early untreated dcSSc skin among CD4+ T cells, TH2 cells are detected along with TH17 cells, follicular helper T cells (Tfh), and regulatory T cells (Tregs). CD4 + CCR7-memory T cells produced IL-13, IL-4, and TNFα, particularly in dcSSc [14]. In addition, IL-13 overproducing CD8+ T cells and IL-4 overproducing CD4 + CD8+ double positive T cells were detected in SSc skin lesions. The role of T-regulatory cells in SSc still conflicting. Most studies have reported that there were decreased frequencies and impaired function of T-regs cells followed by an imbalance of Treg/Th17 with reduced levels of cytokines serum, TGF-β and IL-10. Tregs may act as an anti-inflammatory by releasing cytokines with dual function such as IL-10, thus provide a protective role against atypical immune activation. TGF-β as pro-inflammatory cytokine is involved in Tregs differentiation, but the stimulation is inhibited by Th-1 cytokine, IL-6. The balance between Th17 cells and Tregs is deregulated during SSc development [21–23].

Abnormal T cell activation is a crucial element in the initiation and progression of SSc. The subtle regulation between the interaction of Th1/Th2 cells has long been the focus of the step. Either by releasing soluble mediators like IFN-γ (Th1 cells), IL-4 and IL-13 (Th2 cells), or by directly contacting fibroblasts, Th1 cells are considered anti-fibrotic in inhibiting ECM deposition and promoting MMP secretion, while Th2 cells are the opposite [3, 5, 14]. Fibroblasts respond to fine control of Th1/Th2 cell stimulation, which is followed by secretion of mediator. Th1 cells secrete anti-angiogenic and anti-fibrotic mediators, while Th2 pro-fibrotic and pro-angiogenic. Fibroblasts act as "immune sentinels' in a paracrine manner by releasing cytokines and having direct and indirect cell–cell interactions with immune cells. Continuous two-way communication between immune cells and fibroblasts was thought to be the primary driver of SSc. T cells contribute to endothelial dysfunction and cytokine-mediated macrophage and fibroblast/myofibroblast activation, while fibroblasts secrete ECM, collagens, glycosaminoglycans (GAGs), and fibronectin leading to the formation of fibrosis in SSc. Chizzolini et al. suggested that activated T cells are the dominant lymphocyte population in lesioned skin and in particular T cell infiltrates correlate with skin involvement suggesting an association between autoimmunity and fibrosis [3, 6, 21–23].

T-follicular helper cells were also studied for involvement in SSc pathomechanisms. Several studies have shown higher levels of follicular T cells (Tfh) in peripheral blood and skin, but the remains study has shown inconsistent results. Follicular T helper cells (Tfh) provide essential support for B cell differentiation and antibody production in the germinal centers of secondary lymphoid organs. They express inducible T cell co-stimulator (ICOS), programmed cell death protein 1 (PD) 1, transcription factor BCL6 and produce IL-21 [24]. SSc patients with elevated Tfh cells and plasmablasts more frequently progressed to a late nailfold capillaroscopy pattern that was correlated with internal organ involvement [25]. A recent study showed that early SSc correlated with increased of Tfh cells, particularly SSc with severe skin lesions. Morita et al. in his study reported that there was dysregulation on Tfh homeostasis, identified by increasing cTfh17 and cTh1 cells in SSc patients, associated with the increased plasma level of IL-17F [26]. cTfh17 stimulate pro-inflammatory and pro-fibrotic cytokines, and can induce B cell differentiation, resulting in an imbalance of B cells subsets. Naïve B cells and plasmablast were found increased, while memory B cells were reduced in SSc due to immunologic abnormalities in SSc [27].

Absolute count of B cells shown contradictory result in peripheral blood of SSc patients, as B cells may find decreased, increased, or similar with controls. The different results among these studies might be due to differences methods used, the threshold definition, and/or on treatment of glucocorticoids or immunosuppressants. B cells also contribute to SSc pathogenesis, as specific autoantibodies (ATA, ACA) are found in SSc and B cell secretome includes IL-6 and TGF-β. Increased levels of IL-6 were found in the early diffuse SSc (dSSc), that could stimulate fibroblast from affected skin areas. Therefore, the loop between fibroblast and B cells is partly dependent on IL-6. Other cytokines that were produced by circulating B cells were IL-8, IL-1β, BAFF and CXCL13 (pro-inflammatory cytokines and chemo-attractant).

These cytokines polarized activity of CD4 T cells into Th2, Tfh and/or Th17. Increased of Th2 cytokines then enhanced autoantibody production from plasma cells and contribute to collagen production from fibroblast [28–30].

5. Role of oxidative stress

In SSc, oxidative stress, defined as an imbalance of oxidant and antioxidant states, is generated by fibroblasts, activated leukocytes, dysregulated metabolism of free radical nitric oxide and enhance of isoprostane and nitrotyrosine enzyme that induce oxidative stress, as seen in **Figure 1** [4, 31–33].

A recent meta-analysis on SSc patients described that several biomarkers of oxidative stress were found to be elevated in serum, such as malondialdehyde (MDA), nitric oxide and endogenous nitric oxide inhibitors compared to controls. Increased oxidative stress was also found in urine samples (8-Oxo-2′-deoxyguanosine (8-oxodG) and isoprostanes), lung and skin (increased H_2O_2 and nitric oxide). Fibroblasts extract from fibrotic skins of SSc patients shown higher ROS levels compared to control. These studies suggest that ROS play a role in SSc pathogenesis from earlier state of inflammation on SSc. In endothelial cells, higher levels of hydrogen peroxide were found especially in SSc patients with dcSSc compared to the lcSSc. A study in mice showed that increased levels of H_2O_2 in endothelial cells were able to create neoepitopes that may lead to the production of SSc autoantibodies, anti-DNA topoisomerase I Abs. Other autoantibodies such as anti-peroxiredoxin and anti-methionine sulfoxide reductase A (MRSA) were also detected at higher level in SSc serum. These autoantibodies induced 59% inhibition of peroxiredoxin I enzymatic activity and inactivation of oxidation of proteins by methionine reduction, which leads to chronically increased oxidative stress found in SSc patients. In animal and clinical studies, the local production of hypochlorous acid (HOCl) or hydroxyl radicals can stimulate the immune response and the production of anti-DNA topoisomerase-1 autoantibodies, while the generation of peroxynitrite triggers the production of anticentromere antibodies against centromere protein B. Another study on endothelial cells and fibroblast showed that there was no changes serum-induced ROS production or cell proliferation if autoantibodies were present. However, studies confirm that anti-PDGRF (anti-PDGFR Abs), can trigger the production of ROS and, thus, activate the development of SSc [4, 31–33].

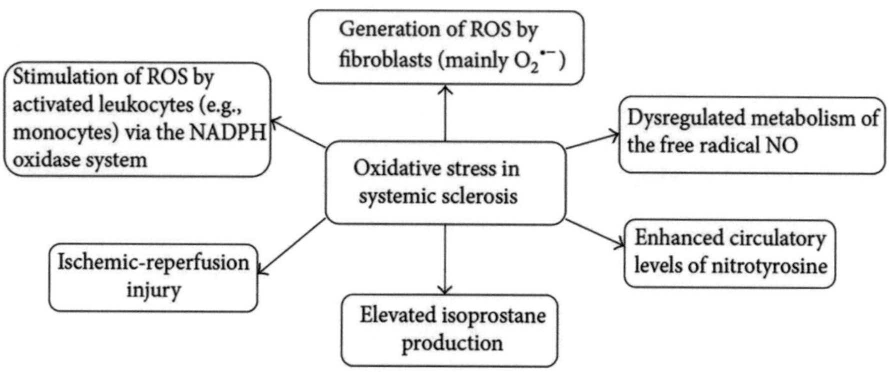

Figure 1.
Patomechanisms of oxidative stress role in systemic sclerosis [4].

6. Inflammasomes in the pathogenesis of SSc

Inflammasomes are large macromolecular cytoplasmic signaling complexes that control the proteolytic activation of two highly pro-inflammatory cytokines, interleukin-1 (IL-1), IL-1B and IL-18 under different signaling from danger to defend the host. Assembly and activation of inflammasomes are triggered by stimulation of the protein recognition receptor (PRR), which interacts with the adapter molecule and is bound to pro-caspase-1. With this caspase-1 is cleaved and activated so it can cleave pro-IL-1B and pro-IL-8, resulting in the active form of IL-1B and IL-8, respectively, which stimulate the inflammatory response. Activation of caspase-1 through the inflammasome pathway is also able to induce pyroptosis, a type of inflammatory cell death [34–37].

Inflammasomes containing the NLR-3 family pyrin domain (NLRP3) are increasingly implicated in many inflammatory conditions. The involvement of NLRP3 on SSc was recognized only recently. The study of the BLM mouse model shows the importance of IL-1B and IL-18 in increasing the fibrosis score. The increase in these cytokines also induced in vivo activation of the NLRP3 inflammasome in a human study. Artlet et al. made a breakthrough by directly linking the upregulation of inflammasomes to the pathogenesis of SSc. In SSc dermal fibroblasts, Artlet et al. found a 5–7-fold increase in NLRP3 inflammasome protein expression, IL-1B, and IL-18, while treatment showed attenuation in levels of collagen and myofibroblast thickness with caspase-1 inhibitor. Upregulation of IL-1B/IL-18 signaling on SSc skin fibroblasts caused an increase in IL-6 and IL-1B 10 times higher after IL-1B treatment compared to fibroblast from healthy control. This result shows positive feedback mechanism and explains why modest initial stimulation might increase in chronic inflammation and subsequent ECM deposition [35–37].

Prolonged exposure of microvascular endothelial cells to IL-1B can induce permanent transformation into myofibroblasts. Chronic inflammation and inflammasomes lead to continuous cleavage of IL-1B in a positive feedback mechanism, which maintains a high level of active TGF-B1 protein, causing fibrosis. IL-18 is also capable of inducing fibroblast proliferation. The first report showing that inflammasomes are involved in SSc pathogenesis was obtained in animal model where IL-1B was shown to be crucial for establishment of bleomycin-induced pulmonary fibrosis. Inflammasomes NLRP3 and AIM2 were found to be increased in SSc lung and skin, while caspase-1 activity is also increased in SSc fibroblasts. SSc lesional fibroblasts secrete more IL-1B and IL-18 with increased clinical parameters of skin thickening suggests a potential role of these cytokines in SSc fibrotic complications.

7. Cytokines as fibrotic mediators in SSc pathogenesis

7.1 Interleukin-1 (IL-1) super family

The IL-1 family of cytokines consists of 11 cytokines, consisting of 7 ligands with agonist activity (IL-1α, IL-1β, IL-18, IL-33, IL-36α, IL-36βand IL-36γ) as well as 4 ligands with antagonistic activity (IL-1Ra, IL-37 and IL-38). Interleukin-1 can also be classified into 3 subtypes, namely IL-1 type 1, type 2 and type 3. IL-1 cytokine members are involved in the innate response and adaptive immunity in SSc, as well as in the process of fibrosis. The IL-1 cytokines that are currently being discussed in connection with SSc are the IL-18 and IL-33. There are not many studies related to the

Common name	Receptor	Potential roles in SSc or fibrosis
IL-1α	IL-1R1	Upregulated in lesional skin and serum. Induce production of IL-6 and PDGF. Promote viability of SSc fibroblasts [38].
IL-1β	IL-1R1 dan IL-1R2	Elevated in the serum, BAL and lesional skin. Induce IL-6 and TGF-B1 and promote Th17 cell differentiation [38].
IL-1Ra	IL-1R1	Upregulated in SSc-affected fibroblasts on skin and lung. Induce fibroblast differentiate into myofibroblast [38].
IL-18	IL-18Ra	Elevated in serum and BAL. Pro-fibrotic and anti-fibrotic effects were reported in fibrosis of skin and lung [38].
IL-33	ST2 (known as IL-1R4)	Downregulated in early SSc and upregulated in late SSc. Elevated in serum. Induce M2 macrophages and ILC2 to produce IL-13 and TGF-B [38].
IL-36	IL-36R	Unknown
IL-37	IL-18Ra	Down-regulate pro-inflammatory cytokines [38].
IL-38	IL-36R	Unknown

Table 1.
Potential role of IL-1 super family cytokines in SSc and fibrosis [38].

role of IL-36, IL-37 and IL-38 in SSc so these three cytokines are still an interesting area for further research [38]. The potential role of the IL-1 superfamily can be seen in the following **Table 1** [38].

Genetic studies of IL-1 in SSc also show that there is a relationship between IL-1 genetic variants and the risk of developing SSc, such as IL-1A, IL-18 and IL-33 variants. The IL-1β variant, SNP rs1143634, is thought to play a protective role in the occurrence of SSc, characterized by the low expression of this variant in SSc patients compared to healthy controls. IL-1 family allele variants and their relation to risk/protection against SSc can be seen in the following **Table 2** [38].

Up to now, IL-1α was the most studied for the involvement in the pathogenesis of SSc from IL-1 cytokine family. Few studies reported that IL-1α is expressed in very high levels in the dermal fibroblasts of SSc patients as compared to normal. In addition, high levels of IL-1α are also associated with the incidence of digital ulcers, which shows a relationship with the incidence of obliterative vasculopathy. IL-1α

IL-1 Family	SNP associated with SSc	Risk/Protection
IL-1A	rs1800587 rs17561	Risk
IL-1B	rs1143634 rs1143627 rss16944	Protection Risk Risk
IL-18	rs1946518 rs187238	
IL-33	rs7044343 rs1157505 rs11792633 rs1929992	Risk

Table 2.
Risk or protection Allel variants of IL-1 super family cytokines [38].

also induces IL-6 which plays a role in the process of fibrosis through pro-fibrotic gene expression in vivo, which increases TGF-B1 production and regulates TGF-B receptors. TGF-B is a major regulatory cytokine of fibrosis through EMT stimulation, fibroblast proliferation, ECM product synthesis and MMP inhibition. IL-1 also induces PDGF, a chemotactic factor that induces the expression of N-cadherin and α-sma, both of which are markers for myofibroblast cells. This further strengthens the role of IL-1α as a cytokine that plays a role in fibroblast-myofibroblast differentiation, myofibroblast longevity which is the main key in the continuation of skin fibrosis in SSc [38–40].

7.2 Interleukin-18 (IL-18)

Interleukin-18 in SSc was found significantly increase compared to healthy control subjects. IL-18 was found to be increased both by serum and BAL examination in SSc with pulmonary disorders, indicating that IL-18 is involved in the fibrotic process that occurs in this disease. The study by Kitasato et al. showed that IL-18 mediates liver cell fibrosis by activating CD4 T cells, which can be suppressed by administration of anti-IL-18. In renal fibrosis, stimulation of the renal tubules with IL-18 can induce a-SMA, collagen-I and fibronectin which stimulate the process of fibrosis. However, another study by Nakatani-Okuda et al. showed opposite results, where IL-18 is also thought to have anti-fibrotic effects. This can be seen from a study they conducted on model mice with IL-18 deficiency, which experienced more severe fibrosis than wild-type mice. Another study by Kim et al. showed that IL-18 down-regulation occurs in human dermal fibroblasts which also indicates an anti-fibrotic effect of IL-18 on SSc, so that the actual role of IL-18 as a pro-fibrotic or anti-fibrotic still requires further research [41, 42].

IL-18 has the capabilities of IL-1 cytokines in general, such as stimulating TGF-B1 expression, inducing type I and type III collagen and mediating collagen gel contraction. In myocardial tissue, administration of IL-18 as a recombinant therapy can lead to remodeling and interstitial myocardial fibrosis [42].

7.3 Interleukin-33 (IL-33)

Elevated serum IL-33 levels are found in SSc and are associated with the severity of skin fibrosis, reduced lung function, and peripheral vascular involvement, such as digital ulcers. An additional study also suggests that IL-33 may be a serum marker for vascular abnormalities in SSc. In the skin biopsies from early SSc patients, the expression of IL-33 protein was down regulated. by contrast, in patients with late stage SSc, IL-33 protein expression was constitutive found in most endothelial cells. Elevated serum IL-33 levels were also found in uterine fibrosis in women and were also found to be elevated by BAL (bronchoalveolar lavage) patients with IPF. IL-33 and its receptor ST2 are increased in fibrotic livers, and they were directly correlated to collagen expression [43, 44].

Studies on IL-33 also show that IL-33 has two types, namely full-length IL-33 and mature IL-33 which are functionally different. Patients with IPF showed a significantly higher increase in full-length IL-33 than mature IL-33. In brief, the critical role of IL-33 in SSc pathogenesis has been elucidating. However, more studies on the precise function of IL-33 in the process of immune dysfunction, vasculopathy, and fibrosis are required in SSc [45].

7.4 TNF superfamily

Although TGF-B is also a major factor in the pathogenesis of fibrosis, it is also known that the TNF superfamily (TNFSF) is involved as a mediator in the inflammatory process. TNFSF is a group of cytokines consisting of 19 ligands and 29 receptors. TNFSF plays a role not only in inflammation, but also in upregulation of the fibrotic process. Several TNFSF ligands are known to be associated with and involved in the process of pulmonary fibrosis, heart, skin, gastrointestinal tract, kidney, and liver [46].

In SSc it is known that the TNFSF involved in pathogenesis are LIGHT, BAFF, OX40L, CD70 and TRAIL which can directly stimulate direct fibrosis in stromal cells (epithelial, fibroblasts and smooth muscle cells). SSc patients are known to have an increase in soluble TNFR1 which is related to the degree of disease severity. Hugle et al. showed that there was upregulation of TNFR1 and TNFR2 in dermal T cells of patients with dcSSc, with TNFR2 being more related to skin thickening [46].

LIGHT is also associated with the risk of pulmonary fibrosis. LIGHT is also found increased? in skin biopsies of patients with SSc [46]. BAFF serum levels are also increased in SSc and can act directly on fibroblast and B cells. OX40L levels are usually associated with the severity or worsening of skin and lung fibrosis, so OX40L is thought to be a marker of fibrosis in the lung [46]. Recent studies have shown that OX40 L can affect the development and progression of fibrosis in various tissues and various degrees of fibrosis severity. CD70 is a ligand that is expressed on antigen-presenting cells (APC) and fibroblast cells. CD27:CD70 co-stimulation is a pathway that activates innate and adaptive immunity in the process of fibrosis because CD27 is expressed more in B cell and T cell subsets. In SSc, CD27 was correlated with the severity of fibrosis in skin biopsies showing that the CD27 pathway: CD70 is an important target for further research. Luo et al. demonstrated that CD70 expression in SSc is related to disease severity, however, further research is needed on the contribution of the CD27:CD70 pathway to the pathogenesis of SSc [46].

TRAIL, also known as TNFSF10, is also known to be associated with SSc, although studies have shown that TRAIL is more related to apoptosis of cancer cells and transformed cells. The results of a study using modified TRAIL as a therapy for skin fibrosis, showed that TRAIL can effectively destroy skin myofibroblasts and can restore the contours of the fibrous skin to close to normal skin in studies with SSc model mice. However, further research is needed to see which sensitive cell types are most associated with TRAIL sensitivity and possibly other pathways that contribute to TRAIL expression [46].

7.5 Interleukin-6 (IL-6) super family

IL-6 is a pleiotropic cytokine that plays a role in the inflammation that underlies SSc disease. IL-6 plays a role not only in the acute phase response, but also in chronic inflammation, autoimmunity, endothelial cell dysfunction and fibrogenesis. The IL-6 cytokine family is a group of cytokines consisting of IL-6, IL-11, ciliary neurotrophic factor (cTNF), leukemia inhibitory factor (LIF), oncostation M (OSM), cardiotrophin-1 (CT-1), cardiothropin- like cytidine (CLC) and IL-27. All of them belong to the same family because of the similarity of their receptor complexes containing the gp130 receptor subunit. IL-6 has a dominant pro-inflammatory activity, through IL-6 trans- signaling activity where IL6-binds to soluble IL-6R(sIL-6R) and then binds to gp130 expressing cell. Some of the effects of trans-signaling activity are the recruitment of MN cells, stimulation of endothelial cells, smooth muscle cells, inhibition of apoptosis by T cells and differentiation of T-reg cells. Meanwhile, classic IL-6 signaling on IL-6R expressing cells provides protective effects including IL-6 dependent regeneration, protection against bacterial infection. Cleaving of IL-6R to form soluble IL-6R is performed majority by ADAM17. In SSc, it is known that ADAM17 has increased activity which initiates the formation of sIL-6R, besides that in SSc there is also an increase in serum IL-8 which stimulates sIL-6R from neutrophils. As IL-6/sIL-6R can bind to the gp130 receptor which activates the STAT3 signal, which in turn increases the expression of the adhesion molecules ICAM-1, VCAM-1, IL-8, and MCP-1 release, accompanied by IL-6 [47, 48].

Interleukin-6 is associated with diffuse skin fibrotic involvement and early disease [49]. SSc patient fibroblasts were also found to express increased IL-6 compared to healthy controls, and IL-6R was also found in skin biopsies of limited cutaneous type SSc. Due to the biological nature of IL-6 trans-signaling, this cytokine can save T cells from cell apoptosis so that it will stimulate chronic inflammatory conditions through a positive autocrine feedback system. The trans-signaling signal is also able to increase autoantigen presentation by suppressing Na+2/K+ATPase by IL-6, it is also suspected that this IL-6/sIL-6R complexion can inapropriately change the signaling pathways of T-cell apoptosis thereby increasing cell persistence. T autoreactive [50].

7.6 Interleukin-17 (IL-17)

IL-17 family cytokines are cytokines expressed by Th-17 cells through the induction of the cytokine Il-23. In the early 2000s, genomic sequencing studies demonstrated that the IL-17 cytokine consists of 6 subtypes namely IL17A, IL17B, IL17C, IL17D, IL17E (also called IL-25), and IL17F. IL-17F is structurally similar to IL-17A (55%), and is more commonly expressed as IL-17A. IL-17B, IL-17C, and IL-17D have a structural similarity of 23–29% with IL-17A, while IL-17E, the most divergent of all IL-17 families, has a structural similarity of around 16%. In IL-17 family of cytokines, IL-17A plays the most important role as a pro-inflammatory cytokine. One of the effect is to maintains the stability of mRNA of TNF induced genes, so that it amplifies the effects of TNF [51, 52].

SSc, characterized by fibrosis of several organs, would be linked to a bias in favor of the activation of immune responses mediated by the Th17 pathway. Studies have shown that IL-17 is significantly higher in the serum of patients with SSc [51]. Increased IL-17A was also found in pulmonary fibrosis, kidney, heart, and skin of SSc patients, and IL-17A was also thought to be related to lung remodeling [51]. Animal studies have shown that IL17A plays a role in skin fibrosis through a TGF-B dependent pathway that induces collagen deposition in skin tissue [52].

Human studies show an increase in IL-17A+ expression in the dermis of the SSc patient skin and this is also followed by an increase in circulating Il-17A [51]. Expression of IL-17A is inversely proportional to the severity of SSc, IL-17A was also found to be associated with SSc fibroblast proliferation but its effects on collagen and ECM protein synthesis are still trivial. In lung tissue, the fibrotic effect of IL-17A has been proven through studies in experimental animals, but studies in humans have not been able to show a clear relationship between IL-17A and the progression of pulmonary fibrosis in SSc patients [51]. Xing et al's study showed that IL-17A in SSc patients mediated endothelial cell inflammation via ERK1/2 phosphorylation. IL-17A can induce endothelial cells which in turn release cytokines and chemokines that activate neutrophil infiltration, also stimulate endothelial cell apoptosis which is thought to be related to endothelial cell dysfunction in abnormal inflammation [52].

DOI: http://dx.doi.org/10.5772/intechopen.1002990

8. Conclusions

SSc, or scleroderma, is a rare and complex autoimmune disease. Research advancement has improved knowledge on how important contribution of inflammation in disease pathogenesis. Oxidative stress leading to inflammatory cells infiltration, activation of ILC and dendritic cells, inflammasomes and Th cells subpopulations disbalance observed in blood and tissue of SSc are the proposed triggering events leading to early endothelial damage which leadsto vasculopathy and vicious circle of extracellular matrix deposition. Dysregulation of innate and adaptive immunity involve several pro-inflammatory cytokines and mediators that regulate fibroblast production of ECM. Several studies proposed the successful treatment of SSc by inhibiting cytokine mediators and inflammasomes, which led to new therapeutic concepts. Future research of these cytokines is warranted to strengthen their role as treatments and biomarkers of SSc in precision medicine.

Author details

Dwitya Elvira* and Raveinal Masri
Division of Allergy and Clinical Immunology, Department of Internal Medicine, Andalas University School of Medicine/M. Djamil Hospital, Padang, West Sumatra, Indonesia

*Address all correspondence to: dwityaelvira@med.unand.ac.id

References

[1] Szabo I, Muntean L, Crisan T, Rednic V, Sirbe C, Rednic S. Novel concepts in systemic sclerosis pathogenesis: Role of miRNAs. Biomedicine. 2021;**9**(1471):1-18. DOI: 10.3390/biomedicines9101471

[2] Benfaremo D, Svegliati S, Paolini C, Agarbati S, Moroncini G. Systemic sclerosis: From pathophysiology to novel therapeutic approaches. Biomedicine. 2022;**10**(163):1-21. DOI: 10.3390/biomedicines10010163

[3] Sepulveda AS, Gonzalez AE, Suarez SA, Lima DE, Islas AE, Castaneda AR, et al. Systemic sclerosis pathogenesis and emerging therapies, beyond the fibroblast. BioMed Research International. 2019;**2019**:1-16. DOI: 10.1155/2019/4569826

[4] Gorniak BG, Puszczewicz M. Oxidative damage and antioxidative therapy in systemic sclerosis. Mediators of Inflammation. 2014;**2014**:1-12. DOI: 10.1155/2014/389582

[5] Suhee K, Park HJ, Lee SI. The microbiome in systemic sclerosis: Pathophysiology and therapeutic potential. International Journal of Molecular Sciences. 2022;**23**(16154):1-23. DOI: 10.3390/ijms232416154

[6] Pattanaik D, Brown M, Postlethwaite BC, Postlethwaite AE. Pathogenesis of systemic sclerosis. Frontiers in Immunology. 2015;**6**(272):1-40. DOI: 10.3389/fimmu.2015.00272

[7] Mitev A, Christ L, Feldman D, Binder M, Moller K, Kanne AM, et al. Inflammatory stays inflammatory: A subgroup of systemic sclerosis characterized by high morbidity and inflammatory resistance to cyclophosphamide. Arthritis Research & Therapy. 2019;**21**(262):1-10. DOI: 10.1186/s13075-019-2057-x

[8] Muangchan C, Harding S, Khimdas S, Bonner A, Barron M, Pope J, et al. Association of C-reactive protein with high disease activity in systemic sclerosis: Results from the Canadian Scleroderma Research Group. Arthritis Care & Research. 2012;**64**(9):1405-1444. DOI: 10.1002/acr.21716

[9] Liu J, Zhang H, Su Y, Zhang B. Application and prospect of targeting innate immune sensors in the treatment of autoimmune diseases. Cell & Bioscience. 2022;**12**(68):1-19. DOI: 10.1186/s13578-022-00810-w

[10] Truchetet ME, Brembilla NC, Chizzolini C. Current concepts on the pathogenesis of systemic sclerosis. Clinical Reviews in Allergy and Immunology. 2021;**2021**:1-22. DOI: 10.1007/s12016-021-08889-8

[11] Frasca L, Lande R. Toll-like receptors in mediating pathogenesis of systemic sclerosis. Clinical and Experimental Immunology. 2020;**201**(1):14-24. DOI: 10.1111/cei.13426

[12] O'Reilly S. Toll-like receptors in systemic sclerosis: An emerging target. Immunology Letters. 2018;**195**:2-8. DOI: 10.1016/j.imlet.2017.09.001

[13] Zhao K, Kong C, Shi N, Jiang J, Li P. Potential angiogenic, immunomodulatory, and anti-fibrotic effects of mesenchymal stem cell derived extracellular vesicles in systemic sclerosis. Frontiers in Immunology. 2023;**14**(112527):1-13. DOI: 10.3389/fimmu.2023.1125257

[14] Mouawad JE, Feghali-Bostwick C. The molecular mechanisms of systemic sclerosis-associated lung fibrosis.

International Journal of Molecular Sciences. 2023;**24**(3):1-14. DOI: 10.3390/ijms24032963

[15] Bhattacharyya S, Midwood KS, Varga J. Tenascin-C in fibrosis in multiple organs. Translational implications. Seminars in Cell & Developmental Biology. 2022;**128**:130-136. DOI: 10.1016/j.semcdb.2022.03.019

[16] Marzeda AM, Midwood KS. Internal affairs: Tenascin-C as clinically relevant, endogenous driver of innate immunity. Journal of Histochemistry and Cytochemistry. 2018;**66**(4):289-304. DOI: 10.1369/0022155418757443

[17] Lemanska-Perek A, Adamik B. Fibronectin and its soluble EDA-FN isoforms as biomarkers for inflammation and sepsis. Advances in Clinical and Experimental Medicine. 2019;**28**(11):1561-1567. DOI: 10.17219/acem/104531

[18] Dhanesa N, Chorawala MR, Jain M, Bhalla A, Thedens D, Nayak M, et al. Fn-EDA (fibronectin containing extra domain A) in the plasma, but not endothelial cells, exacerbates stroke outcome by promoting thrombo-inflammation. Stroke. 2019;**50**:1201-1209. DOI: 10.1161/STROKEAHA.118.023697

[19] Xiong J, Zhao Y, Lin Y, Chen Y, Weng Q, Shi C, et al. Identification and characterization of innate lymphoid cells generated from pluripotent stem cells. Cell Reports. 2022;**41**(5):1-23. DOI: 10.1016/j.celrep.2022.111569

[20] Borgia F, Pomi F, Alessandrello C, Vaccaro H, Gangemi S. Potential role of innate lymphoid cells in the pathogenesis and treatment of skin diseases. Journal of Clinical Medicine. 2023;**12**(3043):1-21. DOI: 10.3390/jcm12083043

[21] Jin W, Zheng Y, Zhu P. T cell abnormalities in systemic sclerosis. Autoimmunity Reviews. 2022;**21**(11):1-10. DOI: 10.1016/j.autrev.2022.103185

[22] Al-Adwi Y, Westra J, van Goor H, Burgess JK, Denton CP, Mulder DJ. Macrophages as determinants and regulators of fibrosis in systemic sclerosis. Rheumatology. 2022;**2022**:1-23. DOI: 10.1093/rheumatology/keac410

[23] Sakkas LI, Bogdanos DP. The role of T cells in systemic sclerosis: An update. Immuno. 2022;**2**(3):534-547. DOI: 10.3390/immuno2030034

[24] Gensous N, Charrier M, Duluc D, Contin-Bordes C, Truchetet ME, Lazaro E, et al. T follicular helper cells in autoimmune disorders. Frontiers in Immunology. 2018;**2018**:9. DOI: 10.3389/fimmu.2018.01637

[25] Wei X, Niu X. T follicular helper cells in autoimmune diseases. Journal of Autoimmunity. 2023;**134**:102976. DOI: 10.1016/j.jaut.2022.102976

[26] Beurier P, Ricard L, Eshagh D, Malard F, Siblany L, Fain O, et al. Tfh cells in systemic sclerosis. Journal of Translational Medicine. 2021;**19**(374):1-9. DOI: 10.1186/s12967-021-03049-0

[27] Ricard L, Jachiet V, Malard F, Ye Y, Stocker N, Riviere S, et al. Circulating follicular helper T cells are increased in systemic sclerosis and promote plasmablast differentiation through the IL-21 pathway which can be inhibited by ruxolitinib. Annals of the Rheumatic Disease. 2019;**78**(4):539-550. DOI: 10.1136/annrheumdis-2018-214382

[28] Beesley CF, Goldman NR, Taher TE, Denton CP, Abraham DJ, Mageed RA, et al. Dysregulated B cell function and disease pathogenesis in systemic sclerosis. Frontiers in Immunology. 2023;**2023**:13

[29] De Luca G, Tomelleri A, Dagna L, Matucci-Cerinic M. The target on B cells in systemic sclerosis. "A midsummer dream" to extinguish inflammation and prevent early disease progression to fibrosis. Clinical Rheumatics. 2021;**40**:2529-2533. DOI: 10.1007/s10067-021-05733-4

[30] Liem S, Neppelenbroek S, Fehres CM, Wortel C, Toes RE, Hulzinga T, et al. Autoreactive B cell responses targeting nuclear antigen in systemic sclerosis. Seminars in Arthritis and Rheumatism. 2023;**58**:152136. DOI: 10.1016/j.semarthrit.2022.152136

[31] Choreno-Parra JA, Cervantes-Rosete D, Jimenez-Alvarez LA, Ramirez-Martinez G, Marquez-Garcia JE, Cruz-Lagunas A, et al. Dendritic cells drive probiotic inflammation and aberrant T cell polarization in systemic sclerosis. Rheumatology. 2022;**2022**: 1-12. DOI: 10.1093/rheumatology/keac489

[32] Moudgil KD, Venkatesha SH. The anti-inflammatory and immunomodulatory activities of natural products to control autoimmune inflammation. International Journal of Molecular Sciences. 2023;**24**(95):1-32. DOI: 10.3390/ijms24010095

[33] Fioretto BS, Rosa I, Matucci-Cerinic M, Romano E, Manetti M. Current trends in vascular biomarkers for systemic sclerosis: A narrative review. International Journal of Molecular Sciences. 2023;**24**(4097):1-33. DOI: 10.3390/ijms24044097

[34] Deuteralou K, Kitas G, Garyfallos A, Dimitoulas T. Novel insights into the role of inflammasomes in autoimmune and metabolic rhemuatic diseases. Rheumatology International. 2018;**2018**:1-10. DOI: 10.1007/s00296-018-4074-5

[35] Lin C, Jiang Z, Cao L, Zou H, Zhu X. Role of NLRP3 inflammasome in systemic sclerosis. Arthritis Research & Therapy. 2022;**24**(196):1-10. DOI: 10.1186/s13075-022-02889-5

[36] Henderson J, O'Reilly S. Inflammasome lights up in systemic sclerosis. Arthritis Research & Therapy. 2017;**19**(20s):1-2. DOI: 10.1186/s13075-017-1420-z

[37] Henderson J, Bhattacharyya S, Varga J, O'Reilly. Targetting TLRs and the inflammasome in systemic sclerosis. Journal of Pharmaceutical Therapy. 2018;**2018**:1-39. DOI: 10.1016/j.pharmthera.2018.08.003

[38] Cavalli G, Colafrancesco S, Emmi G, Imazio M, Lopalco G, Maggio MC, et al. Interleukin-1 alpha: A comprehensive review of IL-1 alpha in the pathogenesis ad treatment of autoimmune and inflammatory diseases. Autoimmunity Reviews. 2021;**20**(102763):1-15. DOI: 10.1016/j.autrev.2021.102763

[39] Xu D, Mu R, Wei X. The role of IL-1 family cytokines in the pathogenesis of SSc. Frontiers in Immunology. 2025;**2019**(10):1-8. DOI: 10.3389/fimmu.2019.02025

[40] Artlett CM. The IL-1 family of cytokines. Do they have a role in scleroderma fibrosis? Immunology Letters. 2018;**195**:30-37. DOI: 10.1016/j.imlet.2017.11.012

[41] Sedimbi SK, Hagglof T, Karlsson MCI. IL-18 in inflammatory and autoimmune disease. Cellular and Molecular Life Sciences. 2013;**13**(919973):1-14. DOI: 10.3389/fimmu.2022.919973

[42] Lin E, Vincent FB, Sahhar J, Ngian GS, Kandane-Rathnayake R, Mende R, et al. Analysis of serum interleukin-1

alpha, IL-1B and IL-18 in patients with systemic sclerosis. Clinical Translational Immunology. 2019;**8**(e1045):1-11. DOI: 10.1002%2Fcti2.1045

[43] Di Carmine S, Scott MM, McLean MH, McSorley HS. The role of IL-33 in organ fibrosis. Discovery Immunology. 2022;**1**(1):1-11. DOI: 10.1093/discim/kyac006

[44] Li L, Zhu H, Zuo X. Interleukin-33 in systemic sclerosis: Expression and pathogenesis. Frontiers in Immunology. 2018;**9**(2663):1-7. DOI: 10.3389/fimmu.2018.02663

[45] Mortafa M, ELShourgbagy EW, Elsaged RA. The role of IL-33 in severity of SSc. Egyptian Journal of Medical Microbiology. 2022;**31**(2):1-5. DOI: 10.21608/ejmm.2022.228611

[46] Steele H, Cheng J, Willicut A, Dell G, Breckenridge J, Culberson E, et al. TNF super family control of tissue remodelling and fibrosis. Frontiers in Immunology. 2023;**14**(1219907):1-24. DOI: 10.3389/fimmu.2023.1219907

[47] John SR. IL-6 family cytokines. Cold Spring Harbor Perspectives in Biology. 2018;**10**(a028415):1-17. DOI: 10.1101/cshperspect.a028415

[48] Metcalfe RD, Putoczki TL, Griffin MD. Structural understanding of IL-6 family cytokine signaling and targeted therapy: Focus on IL-11. Frontiers in Immunology. 2020;**11**(1424):1-25. DOI: 10.3389/fimmu.2020.01424

[49] Zheng B, Keen KJ, Fritzler MJ, Ryerson CJ, Wilcox P, Whalen BA, et al. Circulating cytokines levels in SSc related interstitial lung disease and idiopathic pulmonary fibrosis. Scientific Reports. 2023;**13**(6647):1-7. DOI: 10.1038/s41598-023-31232-4

[50] Kawaguchi Y. Contribution of IL-6 to the pathogenesis of systemic sclerosis. Journal of Scleroderma Related Disorders. 2017;**2**(Suppl2):S6-S12. DOI: 10.5301/jsrd.5000258

[51] Brembilla NC, Senra L, Boehncke WH. The IL-17 family of cytokines in psoriasis: IL-17A and beyond. Frontiers in Immunology. 2018;**9**(1682):1-13. DOI: 10.3389/fimmu.2018.01682

[52] Wei L, Abraham D, Ong V. The Yin and yang of IL-17 in systemic sclerosis. Frontiers in Immunology. 2022;**13**(885609):1-7. DOI: 10.3389/fimmu.2022.885609

Chapter 2

Chromosome Segregation Defects in Scleroderma

Rafael Contreras-Galindo, Souren Paul and Preston M. McCourt

Abstract

Fibrosis in systemic sclerosis (SSc or scleroderma) is characterized by an abundance of chromosome segregation defects and chromosome instability (CIN) that lead to overactivation of autoimmunity and inflammation. This chapter will emphasize the most recent findings on the involvement of centromere and telomere dysfunction in scleroderma. We will discuss how centromere and telomere dysfunction contribute to CIN, fibrosis, and cellular autoimmunity in scleroderma. We will also summarize how chromosome segregation defects in the form of aneuploidy and micronuclei formation activate the Cyclic GMP–AMP synthase (cGAS) Stimulator of interferon genes (STING) pathway of cellular immunity. Activation of this pathway induces production of inflammatory cytokines IFNβ and IL6. Finally, we will summarize the most recent therapies to block the cGAS-STING pathway and treat fibrosis.

Keywords: centromeres, chromosome instability, telomeres, fibrosis, cGAS-STING pathway, micronuclei, IFNβ, IL6

1. Introduction

1.1 Pathogenesis and diagnosis of scleroderma fibrosis

Scleroderma results from increased production and accumulation of collagen and other extracellular matrix (ECM) proteins in body tissues culminating in fibrosis, a thickening of the connective tissue [1]. Fibroblasts, the resident cells of connective tissue are key players of fibrosis in SSc [2]. After tissue damage and immune cell activation, fibroblasts in the ECM differentiate into secretory myofibroblasts in a tissue microenvironment rich in fibroblast growth factor (FGF), transforming growth factor beta (TGFβ), interferon beta (IFNβ) and interleukins 1 and 6 [1, 2]. Buildup of myofibroblasts is responsible for the disproportionate production and accumulation of collagen and ECM proteins in SSc fibrosis [1–4]. Excessive buildup of collagen in the skin, gastrointestinal tract, lungs, kidneys, heart, or other tissues together with microvascular damage and cell-mediated autoimmunity lead to organ dysfunction.

Scleroderma is subclassified into limited cutaneous (lcSSc) or diffuse cutaneous (dcSSc) based on the degree of hardening and thickening of the skin and organ involvement. LcSSc usually affects the skin of the face and lower limbs, while dcSSc affects large areas of the skin and major organs. Although both types of SSc are very incapacitating, dcSSc patients have higher morbidity and mortality due to increased inflammation and fibrosis of internal organs, especially interstitial lung disease (ILD) and heart fibrosis [5–8]. The cause of SSc pathogenesis is yet to be uncovered, although a combination of factors, including immune system dysregulation [8], genetic and epigenetic factors such as mutations in HLA genes [9–11], and reactive oxidizing species (ROS) [12] play a major role. Exposure to environmental factors such as silica, bleomycin, aromatic and chlorinated solvents, ketones, and trichloroethylene have also been linked to the condition in some individuals [2–4, 8, 13–16].

The diagnosis of SSc relies on clinical evaluation and detection of antibodies that recognize the nucleus of the patient's own cells, the so-called antinuclear antibodies (ANAs) [17, 18]. ANAs recognize nuclear components and are detected in as many as 95% of SSc patients [19]. Interestingly, some of these antibodies localize to centromere regions, the middle portion of chromosomes. Anticentromere antibodies (ACAs) were first identified in the lcSSc CREST variant (CREST: calcinosis, Raynaud's phenomenon, esophageal dysmotility, sclerodactyly, and telangiectasia) [20] and served as crucial reagents to study centromere biology. ACAs are found in up to 43% of lcSSc (mostly all cases of CREST), recognize many centromere proteins (CENPA, CENPB, CENPC, and so on, to CENPT), and are associated with a generally more favorable prognosis [20]. However, ACA-positivity is associated with the development of pulmonary arterial hypertension [18–20]. CENPB autoantibodies are present in almost all ACA positive lcSSc patients [21]. CENPB autoantibodies can also be found in Sjogren syndrome and neoplasia [21, 22]. CENPA autoantibodies appear to be more specific for SSc patients at risk of pulmonary vascular disease. Autoantibodies that recognize CENPC alone are associated with Sjogren syndrome and CENPF autoantibodies are associated with cancers [22].

ANAs specific for SSc recognize topoisomerase I, an enzyme that breaks single stranded DNA, relaxes supercoiled DNA, and facilitates chromosome condensation [18]. Antitopoisomerase-I antibodies (ATAs; anti-Scl-70) are mostly found in dcSSc patients (prevalence 20–40%), and correlate with poor prognosis, lung fibrosis, and disease progression [17, 18]. Anti-RNA polymerase III autoantibodies are detected in dcSSc patients (prevalence 10–25%), and serve as markers of rapid disease development and renal crisis [17, 18].

Recent studies have also identified ANAs that localize to telomeres, the protective cap of chromosomes, in 9% of SSc patients [23, 24]. These antibodies recognize the shelterin telomeric repeat binding factor 1 (TERF1) protein and are linked to severe lung disease [23]. Despite their clinical value for specific diagnosis and prognosis of SSc, the etiology of ACAs, ATAs, and anti-telomere antibodies in SSc patients is unknown.

1.2 Centromeres

Centromeres are structural units that modulate the proper division of chromosomes. Destabilization of centromere function results in chromosome instability (CIN), a hallmark of birth defects, cancers, and fibrosis [25–28]. Centromeres have two vital functions; (i) recruit centromere proteins to form the kinetochore, and (ii) keep sister chromatids together before chromosome segregation [29, 30]. Defects in either of these vital functions results in structural and numerical CIN, presented in the forms of lagging chromosomes, dicentric chromosomes, aneuploidy, and micronuclei (**Figure 1**) [31, 32].

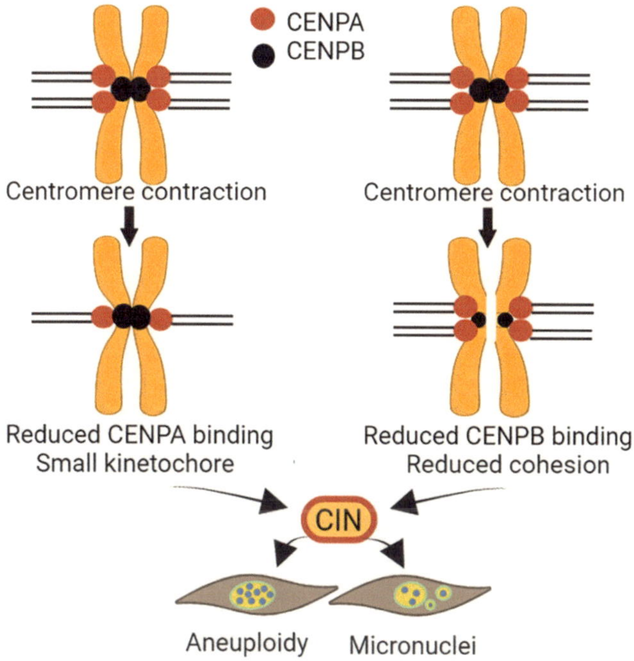

Figure 1.
Centromere function. The H3 CENPA deposits to centromere DNA to initiate the assembly of the kinetochore, which is necessary for microtubule attachment and chromosome segregation. CENPB binds to arrays in the centromere sequence and interacts with CENPA and other centromere proteins to facilitate centromere function. CENPB also binds pericentromere arrays to facilitate chromatid adhesion. Destabilizing these processes, such as centromere sequence deletion or contraction, could reduce CENPA or CENPB binding, leading to CIN. This figure was created with BioRender.com.

Centromere DNA sequences contain arrays of high order repeats (HORs), which can extend several megabases in length (**Figure 2**) [33]. The size of centromere arrays varies among individuals and disease processes. HORs are composed of 171 bp α-satellite units organized in a head-to-tail fashion [33]. During the evolution of hominids, centromeric α-repeats in each chromosome became homogeneous. Today, the α-repeats in each centromere array have 98–100% similarity, yet they have only ~75% similarity to the α-repeats of other centromeres arrays [34, 35]. The centromere core is composed of 1 or 2 arrays [36], while the periphery of the centromeres, the pericentromere, is more diverse, with shorter arrays or monomers of alpha and other repeat types, as well as transposon-like elements [36–38]. Centromeres have been difficult to study because of their repetitive nature, but the genomic assembly of human centromeres has recently been achieved [39–41]. Even so, the human population has a large variation in centromere size and content [41–43].

The function of the centromere is modulated epigenetically by CENPA, a H3-histone variant that forms nucleosomes with H2A, H2B, and H4 at active centromere arrays or elsewhere and defines the location of kinetochore formation (**Figure 2**) [29]. CENPB, a protein that binds to specific DNA sequences in centromeres (CENPB boxes), enhances this centromere chromatin interaction. CENPB interaction with H3K9me3 helps maintain sister chromatid cohesion [30, 44, 45]. Despite the prevalence of ACAs in SSc, the role that centromere sequences and proteins play in the pathogenesis of SSc has remained unexplored.

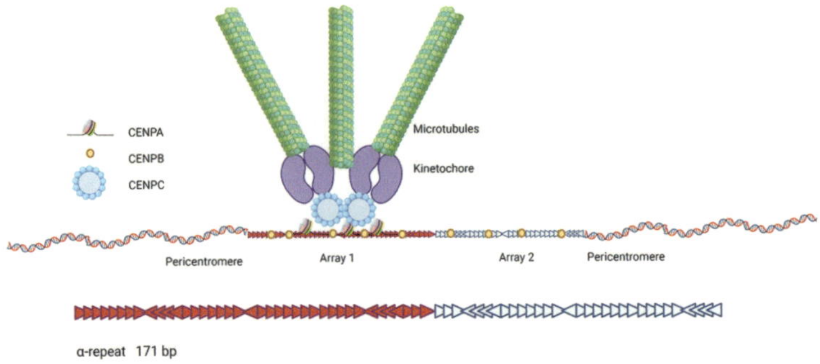

Figure 2.
Organization of human centromeres. Centromere sequences are composed of α-repeats, ~171 bp units, organized in a head-to-tail fashion (arrows). Centromeres sequences are composed of one or two arrays of HORs. Pericentromere sequence contains α- and other satellites. The H3 histone CENPA deposits to the largest array of the core to start the assembly of the kinetochore, which is necessary for microtubule attachment and chromosome replication. H3K9me3 remains abundant at the pericentromeres. CENPB binding to centromere sequences and its interaction with CENPA and CENPC stabilize the formation of the kinetochore. CENPB also binds pericentromere arrays to facilitate chromatid cohesion. This figure was created with BioRender.com.

1.3 Telomeres

Telomeres are specialized chromatin structures that protect chromosome ends. Telomere sequences are regions of TTAGGG repeats that shrink in dividing cells during cell replication [46–49]. The main functions of the telomeres are to (i) protect the terminal regions of the chromosomes from progressive degradation, and (ii) prevent chromosome fusion by ensuring that the DNA repair systems do not mistakenly recognize the very ends of the DNA as DSBs. Excessive telomere shortening or telomere uncapping can produce telomere fusions, which results in CIN, mostly in the forms of dicentric, lagging chromosomes, and micronuclei (**Figure 3**). Telomerase holoenzyme helps maintain telomere length by synthesizing telomeric DNA [46]. Shelterin

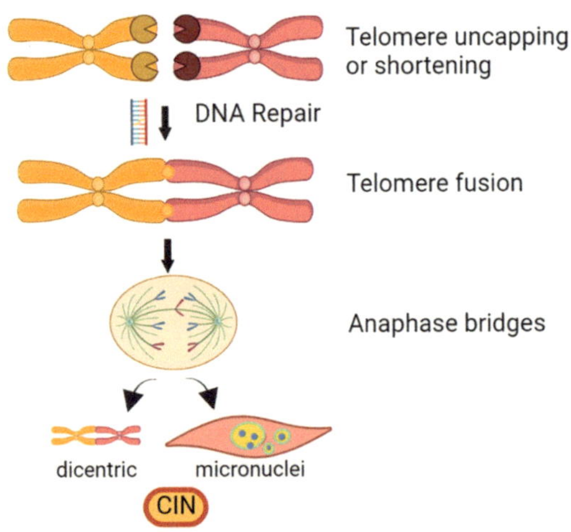

Figure 3.
Telomere function. The telomeric chromatin structure protects chromosome ends from recombination, repair, and fusion. Telomerase holoenzyme counteracts telomere DNA degradation during replication by adding DNA to telomeres, thus preserving telomeres for future cell division. Deletion or degradation of telomeres produces CIN. Recombination and subsequent repair of degraded telomeres can fuse chromosomes, leading to dicentric and/or micronuclei formation. This figure was created with BioRender.com.

complex proteins bind and protect telomeres from degradation and allow access of telomerase and helicase to telomere DNA [46–49]. Although telomerase activity is reduced in somatic cells, it is upregulated in cells that undergo rapid expansion, such as the cells involved in ILD and fibrosis [47, 48]. Thus, it is a distinct possibility that telomerase plays a crucial role in SSc fibrosis.

1.4 Chromosome instability and activation of cGAS-STING/type I interferon pathway

cGAS is an enzyme that senses cytosolic double-stranded DNA from pathogens or damaged self-DNA, such as micronuclei, as part of the innate immune response (**Figure 4**) [50–53]. Upon binding to cytosolic DNA, cGAS produces cGAMP, which interacts with STING to trigger downstream activation of the type I interferon pathway [52, 53]. STING recruits TBK1 to phosphorylate the transcription factor IRF3, which translocates to the nucleus and induce production of type I interferons including IFNβ [53]. Activation of STING also triggers RELA (p65), a component of the NFKB that induces IFNβ and pro-inflammatory cytokines, such as IL6 (**Figure 4**) [49]. cGAS-STING pathway activation is impeded by BANF, which competes with cGAS binding to intracellular DNA, and TREX1, which associates with cGAS and degrades the DNA [54–56]. Fibroblasts from cGAS KO mice do not produce IFNβ following DNA transfection [56]. Aberrant detection of cytosolic DNA has been implicated in cancers and autoimmune diseases [57]. It has also been suggested that cGAS-STING is overactivated in autoimmune diseases such as systemic lupus erythematosus (SLE) [58, 59], and interferons are known to be increased in SSc [60, 61]. Additionally, there are recent findings showing that the cGAS-STING pathway independently triggers fibrosis [62, 63]. As we show below, lesion fibroblasts from SSc patients show increased activation of the cGAS-STING/type I Interferon pathway [64].

2. Chromosome abnormalities in scleroderma cells

Several investigators have noted chromosomal abnormalities in SSc [28, 64–70], including numerical and structural CIN. These findings included micronuclei formation, lagging chromosomes, aneuploidy and polyploidy, chromatid aberrations with gaps and breaks, acentric chromosome fragments, rearrangements, dicentric, and ring forms. These aberrations were specific to lymphocytes, lesion fibroblasts, and bone marrow cells. These cytogenetic abnormalities were more common in advanced forms of SSc, but not in CREST or Raynaud phenomena. Our studies showed increased aneuploidy in forearm lesion skin fibroblasts from dcSSc but not lcSSc patients, which is in agreement with these findings [64]. However, we did not see chromosome abnormalities in lymphocytes or macrophages from the same patients and, the reason for these inconsistencies remains to be clarified. Abnormal nuclear morphology and micronuclei formation were the most common CIN structural abnormalities found in involved skin fibroblasts from SSc patients, suggesting that lagging chromosomes and chromosome fragments failed to be incorporated into the nucleus and were enveloped separately with the nuclear membrane [64, 69, 70]. The clastogenic agent bleomycin further increased micronuclei formation in SSc patient fibroblasts from affected and unaffected skin, but not in skin fibroblasts from healthy controls [69]. The increased chromosomal breakage in dcSSc was not associated with

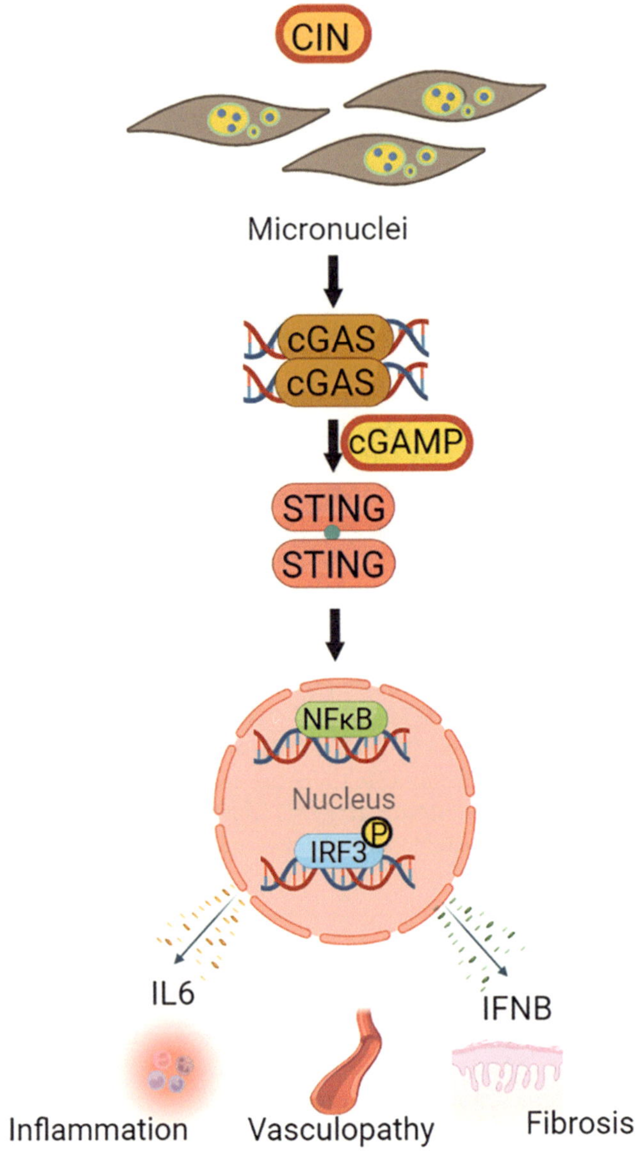

Figure 4.
Function of cGAS-STING pathway. cGAS senses cytosolic DNA from viruses as well as damaged DNA or micronuclei from CIN. Binding of cGAS to cytosolic DNA produces cGAMP, a molecule that interacts with STING to activate the type I interferon pathway. STING activates the expression of NF-κB and phosphorylates IRF3 to induce the production of IL6 and IFNβ, cytokines that mediate inflammation, vasculopathy, and fibrosis.

cancer development or chromosome breakage syndromes [67], although it appears to also be common in SSc family members [65].

3. Centromere defects in scleroderma

Abnormal centromere assembly, localization, and function may lead to errors in chromosome segregation and production of centromere antibodies. Recent studies in our laboratory demonstrated that centromere DNA sequences are shorter at several chromosomes in SSc patients, particularly in lesion dermal fibroblasts [64]. Although changes in the length of centromeres among human populations have been reported [41–43], such dramatic centromere deletion in several chromosomes is pervasive in SSc. Centromere deletions appear to dominate the landscape of several chromosomes in dcSSc, yet centromere arrays in chromosomes 1 and 2 were consistently found deleted in SSc patients [64]. It is unclear why these centromere arrays were particularly deleted, and it is not known whether the deletions contribute to SSc pathology. Further studies indicated these centromere changes were not the result of culture conditions or the previous therapy received by the patients. It remains to be explored whether changes at centromere sequences directly affect the deposition and strength of the kinetochore during chromosome segregation. However, centromere deletions in SSc were found to correlate with abnormal CENPA expression and deposition, which lead to CIN. In fact, SSc fibroblasts show a lack CENPA deposition in micronuclei with CENPB boxes, suggesting that centromere DNA sequences influence centromere function and chromosome segregation as shown in **Figure 1**.

A second important observation was understanding of how centromere changes in SSc patients lead to the production of ACAs [64]. Our studies identified specific centromere defects in lcSSc patients that produce ACAs. Nuclear proteins CENPA and CENPB leaked and colocalized into the cytoplasm and cell membrane of lcSSc dermal fibroblasts. The integrity of the nuclear membrane appears to be one critical factor that contributes to the leaking of centromere proteins, although it is expected that other factors play a role in the specificity of centromere protein misplacement. It remains to be explored what factors, other than rupture of the nuclear membrane, lead to leaking of CENP proteins only in lcSSc patients that produce ACAs. CENPB in the cytoplasm of lcSSc lesion fibroblasts co-localizes with MHC class II molecules DRB1 and DRB5, which suggests a likely mechanism for ACA production in lcSSc [64]. It is possible that the size and complexity in structure of CENPB and perhaps other CENP proteins are more immunogenic. Whether lesion fibroblasts are the sole drivers of aberrant autoimmunity in lcSSc or whether other cell types also act as antigen-presenting cells is unknown.

4. Telomere defects in scleroderma

Studies aimed at understanding the role of telomeres in SSc have found that, similar to centromere deletions, telomere attrition is detected in SSc patients. These recent findings were evident in a subset of SSc patients and telomere shortening was also found to be more prominent in patients with ILD [71, 72]. Whether such telomere deletions also exist in involved skin fibroblasts remains to be studied. Other studies revealed that shorter telomeres in lymphocytes of SSc patients correlated with the production of autoantibodies targeting telomere-associated proteins (shelterin) in a subset of patients. Further, the production of telomere antibodies also correlated with ILD [23, 24]. The recent discovery of telomere autoantibodies in SSc patients may not have been possible before due to the spatiotemporal expression of these proteins and tissue specificity [73]. In contrast, ACAs were discovered in CREST patients even before we understood the structure of centromeres. It is possible that telomere attrition leads to an excess of shelterin proteins that leak to the cytoplasm and act as antigens in a subset of SSc patients. Taken together, these studies suggest that telomere dysfunction affects chromosome segregation and may promote inflammation and fibrosis in SSc as indicated in **Figure 4**.

5. Chromosome instability and cGAS-STING activation in scleroderma and fibrosis

Production of micronuclei and release of DNA into the cytoplasm can activate the cGAS-STING pathway of inflammation and fibrosis [50–53]. Previous reports have shown that SSc fibroblasts produce increased amounts of IL6 and IFNβ, the final molecules activated in the cGAS-STING/type I interferon pathway, although they can be activated by other cellular and immune pathways [74, 75]. Although IL6 and IFNβ may be promising targets to treat SSc, the molecular mechanisms of how these proteins are activated was only recently discovered. The production of IL6 in serum of patients and dermal fibroblasts appears to be specific to SSc clinical phenotypes of dcSSc, such as ILD, pulmonary arterial hypertension, gastrointestinal involvement, and cardiac involvement [76, 77]. On the other hand, increased production of IFNβ and activation of IFN-regulated genes has been observed in the serum and involved skin tissue of patients with SSc [75]. Furthermore, the IFNβ score correlated with markers of disease severity [75]. We observed that increased amounts of micronuclei in SSc dermal fibroblasts strongly correlated with the expression of *cGAS* ($r = 0.6095$), *IFNB* ($r = 0.9562$), *IL6* ($r = 0.5665$), and other-related proinflammatory and profibrotic cytokines [64]. These observations suggest that IL6 and IFNβ are produced by sensing of cytosolic DNA released from micronuclei by cGAS to trigger the cGAS-STING pathway cascade [52]. Increased levels of cGAS colocalized to micronuclei in lesion fibroblasts. cGAS sensing of micronuclei produced increase amounts of 2′3' cGAMP, a second messenger directly produced by cGAS after sensing cytosolic DNA. We further detected the phosphorylation and translocation to the nucleus of downstream factor IRF3, the active Ser-396 phosphorylated form, and detected in the nuclei Phospho p65 (RELA). Finally, we identified the increased IFNβ secretion into the SSc fibroblasts' cell supernatants. Therefore, blocking the cGAS-STING pathway appears to be a promising therapeutic approach to treat SSc. Ex vivo and in vivo studies need to be developed in order to validate this approach and its potential to treat SSc fibrosis.

Although inhibitors of the cGAS-STING pathway have been only examined in autoimmunity in SLE, blocking the final cytokines of the pathway have been explored in SSc. Blockage of IL6 has shown to be promising for reversing the production of TGFβ, a cytokine involved in dermal fibrosis [78]. Further, the efficacy of IL6 inhibitors, particularly Tocilizumab in clinical trials, finishing phase 3, has been satisfactory in preserving lung function, although the primary skin fibrosis endpoint was not met [79, 80]. IFNβ inhibitors per se have been suggested but never studied in SSc [81]. We believe that by blocking the pathway early would prevent the release of both IL6 and IFNβ, attacking the fibrotic and inflammatory component of the disease with a synergistic effect.

We confirmed that cGAS activation was responsible for the IFNβ production in SSc skin cells, treating lesion fibroblasts with G150, a cGAS-specific inhibitor [63]. G150 treatment strongly reduced the cGAS-induced enzymatic (2′3' cGAMP) activity and the production of IFNβ, although the levels of IL6 were not tested. Future research needs to address if cGAS or STING inhibition blocks both cytokines, but also reduces fibrosis of the skin and other organs. Even though current cGAS-STING pathway inhibitors show promising efficacy, they present toxicity to the cells and may harm the body in the long term [82, 83]. Recently, novel CGAS-STING inhibitors have been discovered showing different degrees of specificity for cell types and phenotypes [82, 83]. Therefore, the specificity of new molecules for treating SSc subtypes and phenotypes deserves to be addressed thoroughly for optimal efficacy and safety.

6. Conclusions

We find that telomere and centromere defects at the genetic and epigenetic levels are prevalent in SSc patients and may contribute to chromosome missegregation. Centromere and telomere sequence deletions appear to be important factors that contribute to chromosome segregation defects, and hence, lead to CIN. Such centromere and telomere deletions may have stemmed from ROS or perhaps from exposure to environmental factors that damage the DNA and/or interfere with DNA repair pathways. This review brings to light a new target pathway in SSc, the cGAS-STING/IFNβ pathway, which can contribute to fibrosis. Targeting the cGAS-STING/ IFNβ pathway with newly-developed molecules could prove to be a viable route to treat SSc fibrosis.

Acknowledgements

We are grateful to Drs. David Markovitz, Mark Kaplan, Dinesh Khanna, and Harmit Malik for discussions. R.C-G. was supported by The Hormel Institute, the Rheumatology Research Foundation, an NIH/NCI grant R21-CA259630, and the National Scleroderma Foundation. R.C.-G. is the recipient of the Mark Flapan Award and the Marta Marx Fund for the Eradication of Scleroderma Award from the National Scleroderma Foundation.

Conflict of interest

The authors declare no conflict of interest.

Acronyms and abbreviations

cGAS	Cyclic GMP–AMP synthase
STING	Stimulator of interferon genes
SSc	Systemic Sclerosis
lcSSc	limited cutaneous systemic sclerosis
dcSSc	diffuse cutaneous systemic sclerosis
ROS	reactive oxidizing species
ECM	extracellular matrix
FGF	fibroblast growth factor
TGFβ	transforming growth factor β
IFNβ	interferon beta
IL1	interleukin 1
IL6	interleukin 6
ANAs	antinuclear antibodies
ACAs	anticentromere antibodies

CREST	calcinosis, Raynaud's phenomenon, esophageal dysmotility, sclerodactyly, and telangiectasia
ATAs	antitopoisomerase-I antibodies
DSBs	double-stranded breaks
TERF1	telomeric repeat binding factor 1
CENPB	centromere protein
CIN	chromosome instability
HORs	high order repeats
TBK1	TANK-binding kinase 1
RELA or p65	REL-associated protein
NFKβ	Nuclear factor kappa B
IRF3	Interferon regulatory factor 3
BANF	BAF Nuclear Assembly Factor 1
TREX1	Three Prime Repair Exonuclease 1
SLE	Systemic lupus erythematosus

Author details

Rafael Contreras-Galindo*, Souren Paul and Preston M. McCourt
Hormel Institute, University of Minnesota, Austin, MN, United States of America

*Address all correspondence to: rcontrer@umn.edu

References

[1] Gilbane AJ, Denton CP, Holmes AM. Scleroderma pathogenesis: A pivotal role for fibroblasts as effector cells. Arthritis Research & Therapy. 2013;**15**:215. DOI: 10.1186/ar4230

[2] Katsumoto TR, Whitfield ML, Connolly MK. The pathogenesis of systemic sclerosis. Annual Review of Pathology. 2011;**6**:509-537. DOI: 10.1146/annurev-pathol-011110-130312

[3] Bhattacharyya S, Wei J, Varga J. Understanding fibrosis in systemic sclerosis: Shifting paradigms, emerging opportunities. Nature Reviews Rheumatology. 2011;**8**:42-54. DOI: 10.1038/nrrheum.2011.149

[4] Varga J, Abraham D. Systemic sclerosis: A prototypic multisystem fibrotic disorder. The Journal of Clinical Investigation. 2007;**117**:557-567. DOI: 10.1172/JCI31139

[5] Barnes J, Mayes MD. Epidemiology of systemic sclerosis: Incidence, prevalence, survival, risk factors, malignancy, and environmental triggers. Current Opinion in Rheumatology. 2012;**24**:165-170. DOI: 10.1097/BOR.0b013e32834ff2e8

[6] Elhai M, Meune C, Boubaya M, Avouac J, Hachulla E, Balbir-Gurman A, et al. Mapping and predicting mortality from systemic sclerosis. Annals of the Rheumatic Diseases. 2017;**76**:1897-1905. DOI: 10.1136/annrheumdis-2017-211448

[7] Gabrielli A, Avvedimento EV, Krieg T. Scleroderma. The New England Journal of Medicine. 2009;**360**:1989-2003. DOI: 10.1056/NEJMra0806188

[8] Denton CP, Khanna D. Systemic sclerosis. Lancet. 2017;**390**:1685-1699. DOI: 10.1016/S0140-6736(17)30933-9

[9] Feghali-Bostwick C, Medsger TA Jr, Wright TM. Analysis of systemic sclerosis in twins reveals low concordance for disease and high concordance for the presence of antinuclear antibodies. Arthritis and Rheumatism. 2003;**48**:1956-1963. DOI: 10.1002/art.11173

[10] Tsou PS, Sawalha AH. Unfolding the pathogenesis of scleroderma through genomics and epigenomics. Journal of Autoimmunity. 2017;**83**:73-94. DOI: 10.1016/j.jaut.2017.05.004

[11] Fioretto BS, Rosa I, Romano E, Wang Y, Guiducci S, Zhang G, et al. The contribution of epigenetics to the pathogenesis and gender dimorphism of systemic sclerosis: A comprehensive overview. Therapeutic Advance Musculoskeletal Disease. 2020;**12**:1759720X20918456. DOI: 10.1177/1759720X20918456

[12] Vona R, Giovannetti A, Gambardella L, Malorni W, Pietraforte D, Straface E. Oxidative stress in the pathogenesis of systemic scleroderma: An overview. Journal of Cellular and Molecular Medicine. 2018;**22**(7):3308-3314. DOI: 10.1111/jcmm.13630

[13] Nietert PJ, Silver RM. Systemic sclerosis: Environmental and occupational risk factors. Current Opinion in Rheumatology. 2000;**12**:520-526. DOI: 10.1097/00002281-200011000-00008

[14] Shivakumar DS, Kamath NS, Naik A. Silica associated systemic sclerosis: An occupational health hazard. BML Case Reports. 2023;**16**:e253952. DOI: 10.1136/bcr-2022-253952

[15] Muntyanu A, Milan R, Rahme E, LaChance A, Ouchene L,

Cormier M, Litvinov IV, Hudson M, Baron M, Netchiporouk E; Canadian Scleroderma Research Group. Exposure to silica and systemic sclerosis: A retrospective cohort study based on the Canadian scleroderma research group. Frontiers in Medicine (Lausanne). 2022;9:984907. DOI: 10.3389/fmed.2022.984907

[16] Huang J, Puente H, Wareing NE, Wu M, Mayes MD, Karmouty-Quintana H, et al. STAT6 suppression prevents bleomycin-induced dermal fibrosis. The FASEB Journal. 2023;**37**:e22761. DOI: 10.1096/fj.202200994R

[17] Affandi AJ, Radstake TR, Marut W. Update on biomarkers in systemic sclerosis: Tools for diagnosis and treatment. Seminars in Immunopathology. 2015;**37**:475-487. DOI: 10.1007/s00281-015-0506-4

[18] Kuwana M. Circulating anti-nuclear antibodies in systemic sclerosis: Utility in diagnosis and disease subsetting. Journal of Nippon Medical School. 2017;**84**:56-63. DOI: 10.1272/jnms.84.56

[19] Salazar GA, Assassi S, Wigley F, Hummers L, Varga J, Hinchcliff M, et al. Antinuclear antibody-negative systemic sclerosis. Seminars in Arthritis and Rheumatism. 2015;**44**:680-686. DOI: 10.1016/j.semarthrit.2014.11.006

[20] Song G, Hu C, Zhu H, Wang L, Zhang F, Li Y, et al. New centromere autoantigens identified in systemic sclerosis using centromere protein microarrays. The Journal of Rheumatology. 2013;**40**:461-468. DOI: 10.3899/jrheum.120264

[21] Prasad RM, Bellacosa A, Yen TJ. Clinical and molecular features of anti-CENP-B autoantibodies. Journal of Molecular Pathology. 2021;**2**:281-295. DOI: 10.3390/jmp2040024

[22] Kajio N, Takeshita M, Suzuki K, Kaneda Y, Yamane H, Ikeura K, et al. Anti-centromere antibodies target centromere-kinetochore macrocomplex: A comprehensive autoantigen profiling. Annals of the Rheumatic Diseases. 2021;**80**:651-659. DOI: 10.1136/annrheumdis-2020-218881

[23] Adler BL, Boin F, Wolters PJ, Bingham CO, Shah AA, Greider C, et al. Autoantibodies targeting telomere-associated proteins in systemic sclerosis. Annals of the Rheumatic Diseases. 2021;**80**:912-919. DOI: 10.1136/annrheumdis-2020-218918

[24] Vulsteke JB, Smith V, Bonroy C, Derua R, Blockmans D, De Haes P, et al. Identification of new telomere- and telomerase-associated autoantigens in systemic sclerosis. Journal of Autoimmunity. 2023;**135**:102988. DOI: 10.1016/j.jaut.2022.102988

[25] Verdaasdonk JS, Bloom K. Centromeres: Unique chromatin structures that drive chromosome segregation. Nature Reviews. Molecular Cell Biology. 2011;**12**:320-332. DOI: 10.1038/nrm3107

[26] Yuen KW, Montpetit B, Hieter P. The kinetochore and cancer: what's the connection? Current Opinion in Cell Biology. 2005;**17**:576-582. DOI: 10.1016/j.ceb.2005.09.012

[27] Teh MT, Tilakaratne WM, Chaplin T, Young BD, Ariyawardana A, Pitiyage G, et al. Fingerprinting genomic instability in oral submucous fibrosis. Journal of Oral Pathology & Medicine. 2008;**37**:430-436. DOI: 10.1111/j.1600-0714.2008.00643.x

[28] Emerit I. Chromosomal breakage in systemic sclerosis and related disorders. Dermatologica. 1976;**153**:145-156. DOI: 10.1159/000251109

[29] De Rop V, Padeganeh A, Maddox PS. CENP-A: The key player behind centromere identity, propagation, and kinetochore assembly. Chromosoma. 2012;**121**:527-538. DOI: 10.1007/s00412-012-0386-5

[30] Fachinetti D, Han JS, McMahon MA, Ly P, Abdullah A, Wong AJ, et al. DNA sequence-specific binding of CENP-B enhances the Fidelity of human centromere function. Developmental Cell. 2015;**33**:314-327. DOI: 10.1016/j.devcel.2015.03.020

[31] Krupina K, Goginashvili A, Cleveland DW. Causes and consequences of micronuclei. Current Opinion in Cell Biology. 2021;**70**:91-99. DOI: 10.1016/j.ceb.2021.01.004

[32] Fenech M, Knasmueller S, Bolognesi C, Holland N, Bonassi S, Kirsch-Volders M. Micronuclei as biomarkers of DNA damage, aneuploidy, inducers of chromosomal hypermutation and as sources of pro-inflammatory DNA in humans. Mutation Research, Reviews in Mutation Research. 2020;**786**:108342. DOI: 10.1016/j.mrrev.2020.108342

[33] Liehr T. Microscopic and submicroscopic copy number variations (CNVs) in genetics and counseling. In: Benign & Pathological Chromosomal Imbalances. 1st ed. Amsterdam: Academic Press, Elsevier; 2013. p. 220. DOI: 10.1016/c2012-0-00243-8

[34] Koga A, Hirai Y, Terada S, Jahan I, Baicharoen S, Arsaithamkul V, et al. Evolutionary origin of higher-order repeat structure in alpha-satellite DNA of primate centromeres. DNA Research. 2014;**21**:407-415. DOI: 10.1093/dnares/dsu005

[35] Roizès G. Human centromeric alphoid domains are periodically homogenized so that they vary substantially between homologues. Mechanism and implications for centromere functioning. Nucleic Acids Research. 2006;**34**:1912-1924. DOI: 10.1093/nar/gkl137

[36] Ng TM, Waples WG, Lavoie BD, Biggins S. Pericentromeric sister chromatid cohesion promotes kinetochore biorientation. Molecular Biology of the Cell. 2009;**20**:3818-3827. DOI: 10.1091/mbc.e09-04-0330

[37] Zahn J, Kaplan MH, Fischer S, Dai M, Meng F, Saha AK, et al. Expansion of a novel endogenous retrovirus throughout the pericentromeres of modern humans. Genome Biology. 2015;**16**:74. DOI: 10.1186/s13059-015-0641-1

[38] Contreras-Galindo R, Kaplan MH, He S, Contreras-Galindo AC, Gonzalez-Hernandez MJ, Kappes F, et al. HIV infection reveals widespread expansion of novel centromeric human endogenous retroviruses. Genome Research. 2013;**23**:1505-1513. DOI: 10.1101/gr.144303.112

[39] Jain M, Olsen HE, Turner DJ, Stoddart D, Bulazel KV, Paten B, et al. Linear assembly of a human centromere on the Y chromosome. Nature Biotechnology. 2018;**36**:321-323. DOI: 10.1038/nbt.4109

[40] Miga KH, Koren S, Rhie A, Vollger MR, Gershman A, Bzikadze A, et al. Telomere-to-telomere assembly of a complete human X chromosome. Nature. 2020;**585**:79-84. DOI: 10.1038/s41586-020-2547-7

[41] Nurk S, Koren S, Rhie A, Rautiainen M, Bzikadze AV, Mikheenko A, et al. The complete sequence of a human genome. Science. 2022;**376**:44-53. DOI: 10.1126/science.abj6987

[42] Altemose N, Logsdon GA, Bzikadze AV, Sidhwani P, Langley SA, Caldas GV, et al. Complete genomic and epigenetic maps of human centromeres. Science. 2022;**376**:eabl4178. DOI: 10.1126/science.abl4178

[43] Contreras-Galindo R, Fischer S, Saha AK, Lundy JD, Cervantes PW, Mourad M, et al. Rapid molecular assays to study human centromere genomics. Genome Research. 2017;**27**:2040-2049. DOI: 10.1101/gr.219709.116

[44] Rosandić M, Paar V, Basar I, Gluncić M, Pavin N, Pilas I. CENP-B box and pJalpha sequence distribution in human alpha satellite higher-order repeats (HOR). Chromosome Research. 2006;**14**:735-753. DOI: 10.1007/s10577-006-1078-x

[45] Ohzeki J, Nakano M, Okada T, Masumoto H. CENP-B box is required for de novo centromere chromatin assembly on human alphoid DNA. The Journal of Cell Biology. 2002;**159**:765-775. DOI: 10.1083/jcb.200207112

[46] Shay JW, Wright WE. Telomeres and telomerase: Three decades of progress. Nature Reviews. Genetics. 2019;**20**:299-309. DOI: 10.1038/s41576-019-0099-1

[47] Liu T, Ullenbruch M, Young Choi Y, Yu H, Ding L, Xaubet A, et al. Telomerase and telomere length in pulmonary fibrosis. American Journal of Respiratory Cell and Molecular Biology. 2013;**49**:260-268. DOI: 10.1165/rcmb.2012-0514OC

[48] Arish N, Petukhov D, Wallach-Dayan SB. The role of telomerase and telomeres in interstitial lung diseases: From molecules to clinical implications. International Journal of Molecular Sciences. 2019;**20**:2996. DOI: 10.3390/ijms20122996

[49] Srinivas N, Rachakonda S, Kumar R. Telomeres and telomere length: A general overview. Cancers (Basel). 2020;**12**:558. DOI: 10.3390/cancers12030558

[50] Bai J, Liu F. Nuclear cGAS: Sequestration and beyond. Protein & Cell. 2022;**13**:90-101. DOI: 10.1007/s13238-021-00869-0

[51] Mackenzie KJ, Carroll P, Martin CA, Murina O, Fluteau A, Simpson DJ, et al. cGAS surveillance of micronuclei links genome instability to innate immunity. Nature. 2017;**548**:461-465. DOI: 10.1038/nature23449

[52] Sun L, Wu J, Du F, Chen X, Chen ZJ. Cyclic GMP-AMP synthase is a cytosolic DNA sensor that activates the type I interferon pathway. Science. 2013;**339**:786-791. DOI: 10.1126/science.1232458

[53] Decout A, Katz JD, Venkatraman S, Ablasser A. The cGAS-STING pathway as a therapeutic target in inflammatory diseases. Nature Reviews. Immunology. 2021;**21**:548-569. DOI: 10.1038/s41577-021-00524-z

[54] Guey B, Wischnewski M, Decout A, Makasheva K, Kaynak M, Sakar MS, et al. BAF restricts cGAS on nuclear DNA to prevent innate immune activation. Science. 2020;**369**:823-828. DOI: 10.1126/science.aaw6421

[55] Hemphill WO, Simpson SR, Liu M, Salsbury FR Jr, Hollis T, Grayson JM, et al. TREX1 as a novel immunotherapeutic target. Frontiers in Immunology. 2021;**12**:660184. DOI: 10.3389/fimmu.2021.660184

[56] Fu Y, Fang Y, Lin Z, Yang L, Zheng L, Hu H, et al. Inhibition of cGAS-mediated interferon response facilitates transgene expression. iScience. 2020;**23**:101026. DOI: 10.1016/j.isci.2020.101026

[57] Li T, Chen ZJ. The cGAS-cGAMP-STING pathway connects DNA damage to inflammation, senescence, and cancer. The Journal of Experimental Medicine. 2018;**215**:1287-1299. DOI: 10.1084/jem.20180139

[58] Thim-Uam A, Prabakaran T, Tansakul M, Makjaroen J, Wongkongkathep P, Chantaravisoot N, et al. STING mediates lupus via the activation of conventional dendritic cell maturation and plasmacytoid dendritic cell differentiation. iScience. 2020;**23**:101530. DOI: 10.1016/j.isci.2020.101530

[59] Murayama G, Chiba A, Kuga T, Makiyama A, Yamaji K, Tamura N, et al. Inhibition of mTOR suppresses IFNα production and the STING pathway in monocytes from systemic lupus erythematosus patients. Rheumatology (Oxford, England). 2020;**59**:2992-3002. DOI: 10.1093/rheumatology/keaa060

[60] Fernandez-Ruiz R, Niewold TB. Type I interferons in autoimmunity. The Journal of Investigative Dermatology. 2022;**142**(3 Pt B):793-803. DOI: 10.1016/j.jid.2021.11.031

[61] Vlachogiannis NI, Tual-Chalot S, Zormpas E, Bonini F, Ntouros PA, Pappa M, et al. Adenosine-to-inosine RNA editing contributes to type I interferon responses in systemic sclerosis. Journal of Autoimmunity. 2021;**125**:102755. DOI: 10.1016/j.jaut.2021.102755

[62] Yong H, Wang S, Song F. Activation of cGAS/STING pathway upon TDP-43-mediated mitochondrial injury may be involved in the pathogenesis of liver fibrosis. Liver International. 2021;**41**:1969-1971. DOI: 10.1111/liv.14895

[63] Chung KW, Dhillon P, Huang S, Sheng X, Shrestha R, Qiu C, et al. Mitochondrial damage and activation of the STING pathway Lead to renal inflammation and fibrosis. Cell Metabolism. 2019;**30**:784-799.e5. DOI: 10.1016/j.cmet.2019.08.003

[64] Paul S, Kaplan MH, Khanna D, McCourt PM, Saha AK, Tsou PS, et al. Centromere defects, chromosome instability, and cGAS-STING activation in systemic sclerosis. Nature Communications. 2022;**13**:7074. DOI: 10.1038/s41467-022-34775-8

[65] Emerit I, Housset E, Feingold J. Chromosomal breakage and scleroderma: Studies in family members. The Journal of Laboratory and Clinical Medicine. 1976;**88**:81-86

[66] Wolff DJ, Needleman BW, Wasserman SS, Schwartz S. Spontaneous and clastogen induced chromosomal breakage in scleroderma. The Journal of Rheumatology. 1991;**18**:837-840

[67] Pan SF, Rodnan GP, Deutsch M, Wald N. Chromosomal abnormalities in progressive systemic sclerosis (scleroderma) with consideration of radiation effects. The Journal of Laboratory and Clinical Medicine. 1975;**86**:300-308

[68] Jabs EW, Tuck-Muller CM, Anhalt GJ, Earnshaw W, Wise RA, Wigley F. Cytogenetic survey in systemic sclerosis: Correlation of aneuploidy with the presence of anticentromere antibodies. Cytogenetics and Cell Genetics. 1993;**63**:169-175. DOI: 10.1159/000133527

[69] Martins EP, Fuzzi HT, Kayser C, Alarcon RT, Rocha MG, Chauffaille ML, et al. Increased chromosome damage in systemic sclerosis skin fibroblasts. Scandinavian Journal of Rheumatology. 2010;**39**:398-401. DOI: 10.3109/03009741003685640

[70] Migliore L, Bevilacqua C, Scarpato R. Cytogenetic study and FISH analysis in lymphocytes of systemic lupus erythematosus (SLE) and systemic sclerosis (SS) patients. Mutagenesis. 1999;**14**:227-231. DOI: 10.1093/mutage/14.2.227

[71] Usategui A, Municio C, Arias-Salgado EG, Martín M, Fernández-Varas B, Del Rey MJ, et al. Evidence of telomere attrition and a potential role for DNA damage in systemic sclerosis. Immunity & Ageing. 2022;**19**:7. DOI: 10.1186/s12979-022-00263-2

[72] Lakota K, Hanumanthu VS, Agrawal R, Carns M, Armanios M, Varga J. Short lymphocyte, but not granulocyte, telomere length in a subset of patients with systemic sclerosis. Annals of the Rheumatic Diseases. 2019;**78**:1142-1144. DOI: 10.1136/annrheumdis-2018-214499

[73] Wagner KD, Ying Y, Leong W, Jiang J, Hu X, Chen Y, et al. The differential spatiotemporal expression pattern of shelterin genes throughout lifespan. Aging. 2017;**9**:1219-1232. DOI: 10.18632/aging.101223

[74] Khan K, Xu S, Nihtyanova S, Derrett-Smith E, Abraham D, Denton CP, et al. Clinical and pathological significance of interleukin 6 overexpression in systemic sclerosis. Annals of the Rheumatic Diseases. 2012;**71**:1235-1242. DOI: 10.1136/annrheumdis-2011-200955

[75] Wu M, Assassi S. The role of type 1 interferon in systemic sclerosis. Frontiers in Immunology. 2013;**4**:266. DOI: 10.3389/fimmu.2013.00266

[76] Lin X, Ding M, Chen T, Min S, Wang D, Jiang G. Peripheral blood IL-6 levels in systemic sclerosis patients: Correlation between IL-6 levels and clinical phenotypes. Journal of Cosmetic Dermatology. 2022;**21**:6086-6091. DOI: 10.1111/jocd.15133

[77] O'Reilly S, Cant R, Ciechomska M, van Laar JM. Interleukin-6: A new therapeutic target in systemic sclerosis? Clinical Translational Immunology. 2013;**2**(4):e4. DOI: 10.1038/cti.2013.2

[78] Denton CP, Ong VH, Xu S, Chen-Harris H, Modrusan Z, Lafyatis R, et al. Therapeutic interleukin-6 blockade reverses transforming growth factor-beta pathway activation in dermal fibroblasts: Insights from the faSScinate clinical trial in systemic sclerosis. Annals of the Rheumatic Diseases. 2018;**77**:1362-1371. DOI: 10.1136/annrheumdis-2018-213031

[79] Bohdziewicz A, Pawlik KK, Maciejewska M, Sikora M, Alda-Malicka R, Czuwara J, et al. Future treatment options in systemic sclerosis-potential targets and ongoing clinical trials. Journal of Clinical Medicine. 2022;**11**:1310. DOI: 10.3390/jcm11051310

[80] Khanna D, Lin CJF, Furst DE, Goldin J, Kim G, Kuwana M, et al. Tocilizumab in systemic sclerosis: A randomised, double-blind, placebo-controlled, phase 3 trial. Lancet. Respiratory Medicine. 2020;**8**:963-974. DOI: 10.1016/S2213-2600(20)30318-0

[81] Kakkar V, Assassi S, Allanore Y, Kuwana M, Denton CP, Khanna D, et al. Type 1 interferon activation in systemic sclerosis: A biomarker, a target or the culprit. Current Opinion in Rheumatology. 2022;**34**:357-364. DOI: 10.1097/BOR.0000000000000907

[82] Guerini D. STING agonists/antagonists: Their potential as therapeutics and future developments. Cell. 2022;**11**:1159. DOI: 10.3390/cells11071159

[83] Li Q, Tian S, Liang J, Fan J, Lai J, Chen Q. Therapeutic development by targeting the cGAS-STING pathway in autoimmune disease and cancer. Frontiers in Pharmacology. 2021;**12**:779425. DOI: 10.3389/fphar.2021.779425

Chapter 3

What Comes before Scleroderma?

Silvia Bellando-Randone, Yossra Suliman, Sana Anwar and Daniel E. Furst

Abstract

While the classification criteria for systemic sclerosis (SSc) have been carefully delineated, the definition of what comes before meeting classification criteria is not so well understood. In some ways, it is similar to "pre-rheumatoid arthritis" where a reasonable definition has been developed and the downstream early treatment of "pre-rheumatoid arthritis" is being tested. However, for SSc, there may well be a very early SSc phase before any, but constitutional symptoms occur. This preclinical phase is very poorly understood or described. The very early diagnosis of systemic sclerosis (VEDOSS) has been defined, but there remain multiple questions surrounding VEDOSS, including when and how to treat patients with this diagnosis. Despite progress, there are no fully validated biomarkers or genetic predictors for disease evolution. Moreover, although VEDOSS patients with Raynaud's phenomenon (RP), autoantibodies and SSc capillaroscopic pattern could be easily followed up, and no targeted cohort study to achieve these ends has been developed. Such a cohort study is very much needed, but it would require documenting all appropriate clinical, genetic, and autoimmune measures, followed for at least 5 and perhaps more years, using a randomized menu of treatments.

Keywords: pre-scleroderma, pre-RA, VEDOSS, scleroderma, scleroderma sine scleroderma

1. Introduction

1.1 Personalized or precision medicine

The use of the term "precision medicine" has recently become increasingly popular as has "personalized medicine". They conceptualize the combination of individualized clinical, laboratory, imaging, and genetic data, to fit a specific treatment to a specific patient [1]. This is particularly useful in the management of complex and heterogeneous diseases such as rheumatoid arthritis (RA) or systemic sclerosis (SSc) in which advances in the identification of epigenomic, transcriptomic, and proteomic factors that change during the progression of these diseases or in response to treatment have increased their application for optimal patient management.

1.2 Outline

This chapter first gives the background regarding pre-connective tissue disease. Next, it uses rheumatoid arthritis as an example of the successful use of this concept. Thereafter, the chapter examines pre-scleroderma and very early diagnosis of systemic sclerosis (VEDOSS) and their potential in the future treatment of scleroderma.

2. Background

2.1 Early diagnosis of SSc

Despite knowing that classification criteria are not diagnostic criteria, such classification criteria are regularly used for diagnosis. Several attempts have been made over the years to overcome the diagnostic delay due to the clinical use of the American College of Rheumatology (ACR) 1980 classification criteria, as diagnostic criteria. These criteria require, as a major criterion, skin involvement for identifying SSc patients and starting to treat them. It is of note that skin thickening has been identified as the hallmark of SSc and has unintentionally led to relatively late diagnosis. This was because sufficient skin involvement to meet these classification criteria (1980) often occurred only after several years of disease and after visceral involvement has occurred, dooming clinical trials and effective treatment.

2.2 Typical elements of very early SSc

The recent identification of some typical elements of the very early stages of SSc, named as "red flags," with various combinations of Raynaud's phenomenon (RP), positive anti-nuclear antibodies (ANA), puffy fingers, abnormal nailfold capillaroscopy, and SSc specific antibodies [2], has shifted attention toward patients with SSc characteristics prior to classic skin thickening.

2.3 Problems inherent to the present SSc diagnosis

Unfortunately, these measures, while sensitive, are not highly specific [3] (sensitivity: 0.75; specificity: 0.72) [4]. Given this lack of specificity, it would be necessary to generate a better prediction model about the likelihood that patients will develop SSc. In 2013, the SSc ACR/EULAR (American College of Rheumatology/European Alliance for Rheumatology) classification criteria [5] were published, demonstrating increased sensitivity and specificity, (sensitivity: 0.91; specificity: 0.92) compared to ACR 1980 SSc classification criteria, not absolutely requiring skin fibrosis. These classification criteria resulted in earlier diagnosis of SSc, creating a "window of opportunity" for earlier treatment before significant visceral involvement or damage has occurred.

3. Introduction to pre-RA

It may be asked why should a section on rheumatoid arthritis be in a chapter on SSc? The issue of pre-RA is the one which has been well researched and much is known about its implications. Therefore, examining and understanding "pre-RA" is a template for considering "pre-SSc" and may lead to a better understanding of whether "pre-SSc" exists and what might be done to treat if it does.

The concept of "Pre-RA" is well known. This is a disease stage in which classification criteria are not yet met but the probability of developing RA is high. While the specifics of this "pre-RA" diagnosis have changed over time, the basic concept is to treat prior to significant symptomatic disease and prevent progression to classification/diagnostic criteria, thus preserving the quality of life and preventing long-term anatomic deterioration [6].

3.1 Characterizing "pre-RA"

The term "pre-RA" applies to events that occur prior to the clinical onset of RA as defined by ACR/EULA, classical [7] or during an asymptomatic phase [8, 9]. It is marked, however, by abnormal immune function and responses, even in the absence of clinical signs of autoimmune tissue injury [10].

Several factors in addition to clinical factors contribute to the different fates of patients presenting with apparently similar characteristics. There are genetic predispositions, such as the human leukocyte antigen (HLA) DR genotypes, environmental factors, such as smoking, and serological characteristics (cyclic citrullinated peptide (CCP) and rheumatoid factor) [11].

Rheumatoid arthritis has a preclinical period during which genetic and environmental factors interact, possibly in a sequential manner, to initiate and propagate the autoimmune process, leading to tissue inflammation and injury. During this period, disease-related autoantibodies, such as rheumatoid factor (RF) and anti-citrullinated peptide antibodies (ACPA), can develop even in the absence of clinical signs and symptoms of tissue injury. At a later stage, some but not all patients may experience minimal symptoms or signs that are considered nonspecific or unclassifiable for any rheumatic disease [11].

The EULAR study group recommends that, in prospective studies, individuals at risk of developing RA should be described as having the following five stages [12–14].

1. Genetic risk factors for RA

2. Environmental risk factors for RA

3. Autoimmunity associated with RA

4. Symptoms without clinical evidence of arthritis

5. Unclassified arthritis

3.1.1 Genetic risk factors

The shared epitope refers to a conserved amino acid sequence within the antigen-binding groove of the HLA-DRB1 molecule. In Caucasians, this sequence is present in several HLA-DRB1 alleles, including *0401, *0404, *0405, *0408, *0410, *0413, *0416, *0419, and *0421. These alleles share a common amino acid motif at positions 70 to 74 (Q/R-K/R-R-A-A)*. The increased risk of RA associated with HLA has an odds ratio of approximately 6, in Caucasians. Also, a family history of RA increases the risk of disease by 3 to 10 times [15, 16].

3.1.2 Environmental risk factors

Several environmental risk factors have been identified that contribute to the susceptibility of developing rheumatoid arthritis (RA). These factors include the following.

3.1.2.1 Smoking

Smokers have a higher risk of developing RA, and smoking also tends to worsen the disease progression and response to treatment. For example, smokers carrying two HLA-SE copies face a 40-fold increased risk of RA, highlighting the interplay of genetic and environmental factors in its development. Moreover, the risk remains elevated for up to 20 years after quitting smoking [17].

3.1.2.2 Infections

Chronic periodontal disease (periodontitis) has been linked to a higher risk of developing RA. Martinez-Martinez et al. found periodontal bacterial DNA in all synovial fluid samples and 83.5% of serum samples from RA patients. Despite this, synovial fluid samples from RA patients did not yield bacterial growth, and bacterial DNA was not identified in leukocytes [18].

Additionally, some bacterial and viral infections, such as *Porphyromonas gingivalis* (*P. gingivalis*), *Proteus mirabilis* (*P. mirabilis*), Epstein-Barr virus (EBV), and mycoplasma, have been implicated as potential triggers of RA in susceptible individuals [19]. A study indicates that individuals with elevated serum IgG antibody levels against early antigen of EBV, even if the antibody is found in the preclinical phase, are likely to develop RA. This implies, increased EBV reactivation cycles during this phase [20].

3.1.2.3 Obesity

Adipose tissue produces pro-inflammatory molecules that contribute to chronic inflammation and adiponectin (released by fat cells) levels in RA. Hyperlipidemia linked to obesity plays a role in RA development, particularly in women. Obesity, leads to increase in RA susceptibility through metabolic and endocrine pathways [21]. This involves elevated secretion of proinflammatory cytokines and adipokines by adipocytes, along with disturbances in sex hormone metabolism, resulting in heightened estrogen levels due to increased aromatase activity in adipose tissue [22]. Although some studies diverge, most affirm a link between adiponectin and inflammation markers like CRP. Recent research also associates adiponectin with C-reactive protein (CRP) levels and confirms a positive correlation with the DAS28 disease activity score [21, 23].

3.1.2.4 Hormonal factors

In investigating RA development, numerous studies have explored hormonal factors. A higher occurrence of RA in women compared to men (2 to 3:1) peaks at menopause. Although not well understood, it is believed that hormones may influence the immune response and contribute to the development of RA [24].

3.1.2.5 Dietary factors

While the relationship between diet and RA is complex, some dietary factors have been studied in relation to RA risk. For example, omega-3 fatty acids found in certain fish and plant sources have an anti-inflammatory effect. Kremer et al. carried out controlled studies, showing that greater than or equal to 3.0 g omega-3 acids (found in abundance in fish) had a mild anti-inflammatory effect [25]. On the other hand, diets high in red meat and processed foods have been associated with an increased risk of RA [26].

These environmental risk factors do not directly cause RA but rather contribute to the overall risk of this disease and may interact with genetic factors to trigger the development of the disease.

3.2 Serological precursors of pre-RA

Serological precursors of pre-rheumatoid arthritis can help in identifying individuals who may progress to RA. Here are some important serological precursors associated with pre-RA.

3.2.1 Rheumatoid factor (RF)

Rheumatoid factor (RF) can be detected in pre-RA individuals [27]. For example, among 79 patients with RA who were blood donors and had pre-RA samples, rheumatoid factor has the positive medium of 4.5 years (range: 0.1–13.8) before diagnosis [28].

3.2.2 Anti-cyclic citrullinated peptide antibodies

Anti-cyclic citrullinated peptide antibodies (anti-CCP target proteins that have undergone citrullination): Anti-CCP antibodies are highly specific (85–99% specific when found) for RA and are often present in pre-RA individuals [29, 30]. Studies have shown that individuals who are positive for anti-CCP antibodies have a 20–70% chance of developing RA within 2 to 5 years [29, 31–33].

Its presence is sensitive, but nonspecific and tends to occur more proximate to the appearance of clinical symptoms, usually appearing, within 1 year of clinical disease. However, 40% of RA patients have normal levels. In a large observational study of over 9000 patients, 26% had discordant ESR and CRP, making them unreliable for predicting joint damage progression [34, 35].

3.2.3 Other autoantibodies

Besides RF and anti-CCP antibodies, can be present in the blood of pre-RA individuals. These include anti-carbamylated protein antibodies (anti-CarP) and anti-mutated citrullinated vimentin antibodies (anti-MCV) [36]. Their presence may indicate an increased risk of developing RA. A recent study found a 42% sensitivity and 96% specificity of anti-CarP in anti-CCP and RF-negative RA patients [37].

It should be remembered that the presence of these serological precursors does not guarantee that an individual will develop RA. However, their detection can help identify individuals who may benefit from closer monitoring and early intervention to prevent or minimize the progression of the disease.

3.3 Diagnosing pre-RA

Compared to rheumatoid factor (RF), anti-CCP antibodies seem to provide a better prediction model for future RA development. When both RF and anti-CCP are found together, the hazard ratio of developing RA is 2.87 (1.22–6.76) [30–32, 38]. The wide range of the confidence interval reflects the variability of disease progression among different individuals.

3.3.1 Additional factors

To improve the accuracy of prediction, additional factors can be considered. Certain genetic factors, such as the presence of specific human leukocyte antigen (HLA) alleles such as those noted above, can further increase the risk of developing RA. The presence of the HLA-DRB1 shared epitope is highly correlated with anti-CCP-positive RA development. HLA-DRB1 SE alleles are much more common in patients with anti-CCP (82–89.6%) compared to those without (53–70%). Additionally, the presence of other symptoms related to arthritis, even in the absence of clearly inflamed joints upon physical examination, can be considered when assessing the likelihood of progression to RA [39].

3.4 Using pre-RA to consider therapy

The PRAIRI study, which investigated the effects of rituximab versus placebo in anti CCP- and RF-positive individuals who did not have RA, but might have had arthralgias, demonstrated a delay in the onset of arthritis by approximately 12 months for those who received rituximab [40]. This suggests that targeted interventions have the potential to prevent or delay the development of full-blown RA [41]. Currently, there are several studies, in the pre-RA period to prevent or delay the onset of RA. These studies investigated drugs like methotrexate and abatacept as potential interventions [40–42].

These tests and predictive models provide the probability of a patient progressing to RA but are not infallible. Clinical history, examination, understanding of social situations, etc. (i.e., clinical judgment) are also necessary before embarking on treatment "and no treatment is without at least potential adverse effects" including hepatotoxicity, birth defects, heightened infection risk, lymphoma, and increased skin cancer risk. Regular monitoring is crucial during RA treatment.

Summary: The extensive research done in pre-RA is worth reviewing as it provides the template when considering pre-SSc. Thus, when considering pre-SSc, some factors to consider might include genetics, the environment (e.g., smoking and hormonal factors), antibodies, and autoantibodies which could make diagnosing pre-SSc and its therapy practical.

4. Characterizing SSc

The concept of personalized medicine in SSc is to identify precise predictors of disease that can be targeted to either prevent or significantly delay the onset of clinical SSc. The above considerations in pre-RA can sometimes be applied below.

4.1 Clinical characterization

SSc is an unpredictable autoimmune disease with a high rate of morbidity and mortality as well as high socioeconomic costs because it has a chronic and debilitating course [43, 44]. This disease can be devastating and have a profound impact on quality of life and life expectancy., with a standardized mortality ratio of 3.5 [45, 46]. The great heterogeneity of Refs. [47–49] both clinical manifestations at the onset and during disease evolution requires looking for potential predictors starting from its preclinical and asymptomatic phases (very early SSc). This, in turn, requires the development of effective personalized/precision medicine strategies, one of which is the discovery, and use of SSc biomarkers, that can be identified early before the onset of skin fibrosis and organ damage.

4.2 Response to treatment

Despite presenting with similar initial clinical symptoms, SSc patients often exhibit varying responses to treatment with a standardized mortality ratio of 3.5 [45, 46]. Patients primarily experiencing an inflammatory phase may benefit from immunomodulatory treatments, while those in the fibrotic phase may require anti-fibrotic interventions. In cases where patients exhibit a combination of fibrosis and inflammation, combination therapy may be necessary. Moreover, the majority of patients need vasoactive therapies, beginning during the very early phases of the disease because they have Raynaud's phenomenon (RP) and vascular impairment.

This multiplicity of pathways requires the administration of appropriate therapies targeting the underlying disease mechanistic pathways in a timely manner. Ultimately, targeting such pathways may halt/delay SSc disease progression. Having in mind such a preventive rationale, may pave the way for more innovative medications/approaches in certain SSc phenotypes. By integrating molecular characteristics with clinical phenotypes, innovative and more detailed stratification systems could significantly improve therapeutic approaches in personalized medicine, ultimately leading to better patient outcomes.

The great heterogeneity of SSc manifestations [47] at the onset and during disease evolution requires one to look for potential predictors of SSc starting from its pre-clinical and asymptomatic phases (very early SSc). This, in turn, requires the discovery and validation of SSc biomarkers that can be identified early, before the onset of clinical manifestations.

4.3 Autoantibodies

SSc-specific autoantibodies, including anti-centromere (ACA), anti-topoisomerase (ATA (ScL-70)), and anti-RNA polymerase III antibody (anti-RNAP III), are markers of disease progression and internal organ involvement [50]. These autoantibodies, which are commonly observed in SSc patients, typically occur independent of each other (**Table 1**). Unfortunately, the use of autoantibodies only contributed a small amount to effective risk stratification [51]. A cluster analysis, utilizing a large database and considering clinical and serologic variables from 120 EUSTAR centers (comprising 6927 patients), revealed that the dichotomous classification of SSc patients as lcSSc or dcSSc was insufficient. A significant proportion of lcSSc patients (39%) and dcSSc patients (19%) clustered in a discordant manner. To overcome this limitation, the study incorporated data in the presence of organ damage to predict the risk of further organ damage or death. As a result, the study identified six different clusters characterized by more homogeneous clinical phenotypes [52].

4.4 Pre SSc

4.4.1 Molecular stratification (monocyte sub setting)

The monocyte subset was incorporated by van der Kroef et al. [53]. In SSc characterization, they reported that prior to the onset of skin fibrosis and other organ

Clinical stratification and antibody profile of each cluster [52]
Cluster 1 (1186 pts): female, older onset, GI involvement, lcSSc, ACA (less ILD) Cluster 2 (720 pts): ILD, PH, lcSSc, ACA, ATA Cluster 3 (1243 pts): younger onset, lowest mRSS, less aggressive, lcSSc, ACA > ATA Cluster 4 (1673): older onset, DU, cardiac, lung, MSK, GI involvement, lcSSc, ATA > ACA Cluster 5 (1249): male, younger onset, multi-organ involvements (cardiac, lung, GI, joint), dcSSc, ATA > ACA Cluster 6 (856 pts): male, youngest onset, most aggressive, multi-organ involvement (cardiac, lung, renal, GI, MSK), dcSSc, ATA
Scleroderma-antibodies distinctive clusters [50]
ACA: lcSSc, PAH ATA: dcSSc, ILD anti-RNAP III: lcSSc, SRC anti-PM-Scl: PM/DM overlap, arthritis overlap, ILD anti-Th/To: lcSSc, ILD, PAH anti-Ku: muscle and joint involvement anti-U1RNP: overlap syndromes anti-U3RNP: dcSSc, muscle involvement, PAH anti-U11/U12RNP: ILD
Monocyte subsetted clusters [53]
Cluster 1 (high CD16+ monocyte, low memory B-cell subsets): more in lcSSc Cluster 2 (high classical monocytes): dcSSc, high mRSS Cluster 3 (high memory B cells): usually showed less skin involvement Cluster 4 (low classical monocytes): usually showed less skin involvement

lc, limited cutaneous; dc, diffuse cutaneous; ACA, anti-centromere antibody; ATA, anti-topoisomerase antibody; ANA, anti-nuclear antibody; SSc, systemic sclerosis; Ab, antibody; ILD, interstitial lung disease; PAH, pulmonary arterial hypertension; PH, pulmonary hypertension; RP, Raynaud's phenomenon; SRC, scleroderma renal crisis; PM, polymyositis; DM, Dermatomyositis; NFC, nailfold capillaroscopy; MSK, musculoskeletal; GI, gastrointestinal; mRSS, modified Rodnan skin score; DU, digital ulcer.

Table 1.
Proposed classification systems in systemic sclerosis based on published studies.

manifestations, patients with RP, SSc-specific autoantibody positivity, and/or specific nailfold video capillaroscopy (NVC) patterns exhibited distinct frequencies of immune cell subsets. Through cluster analysis, it was demonstrated that circulating immune cell populations could differentiate SSc subsets into four distinct clusters: cluster 1 (characterized by high CD16+ monocytes and low memory B cells), cluster 2 (showing increased classical monocytes), cluster 3 (exhibiting increased memory B cells), and cluster 4 (displaying lower classical monocytes) [53]. These clusters were associated with different clinical features, such as limited cutaneous involvement in cluster 1, no skin involvement in clusters 3 and 4, and an enrichment of patients with ILD and diffuse cutaneous involvement in cluster 2. Mankinde et al. took a slightly different approach. Using an early SSc data registry and unbiased cluster analysis of monocytes, they found a stable transcriptional signature among three monocyte subsets. Although there were no differences in skin involvement among groups A, B, and C, at baseline, groups B and C had worse lung involvement [54].

4.4.2 SSc gene signature phenotyping

Gene signature phenotyping identified three main intrinsic gene subsets: fibroproliferative, inflammatory, and normal-like. Serial skin biopsies demonstrated that these intrinsic gene subsets were inherent and stable features of the disease in a given patient, indicating distinct pathogenic processes among SSc patients [55, 56]. A recent study by Skaug et al. [57] further reported that immune cell and fibroblast signatures in early dcSSc changed over time, showing a trend toward normalization as these signatures declined during follow-up. This finding has implications for patient stratification in future clinical trials focusing on early-stage disease. The intrinsic gene subsets were consistently observed across different skin biopsy sites, regardless of clinical involvement (thickened or normal skin) [58, 59]. Furthermore, these intrinsic gene subsets were found to be conserved across tissues such as the esophagus and skin, highlighting shared pathogenic processes in SSc across different tissues. However, the issue of microenvironment may influence gene expression, as functional genomic network analysis conducted by Taroni et al. identified a distinct lung-specific innate immune process, indicating that certain gene pairs are more likely to interact in specific tissues compared to others [58, 59].

4.5 Very early diagnosis of systemic sclerosis (VEDOSS)

Previously, in SSc, various terms have overlapped, that is, "early SSc," "VEDOSS," pre-scleroderma, and undifferentiated connective tissue disease (UCTD) at risk for systemic sclerosis (UCTD-risk-SSc) [44, 48, 49, 60, 61]. These terms may identify different clinical scenarios that have something in common and are positioned in the very early phase of SSc. In fact, the term pre-SSc today identifies a moment in time where the disease may be represented by the presence of vague symptomatology (e.g., fatigue) with/without Raynaud's phenomenon (RP) and specific antibodies only. Clearly, having only RP does not mean that SSc already exists, but the presence of specific antibodies, with or without RP, should raise the suspicion that the patient will develop VEDOSS or definite SSc. Its usefulness for diagnostic purposes is limited due to its low specificity as RP may also be found in other connective tissue diseases such as mixed connective tissue disease (MCTD), undifferentiated connective tissue disease (UCTD), systemic lupus erythematosus (SLE), dermatomyositis/polymyositis, Sjögren's syndrome (SS), vasculitis, and RA [62–65]. The latency between RP and the onset of the first non-RP-symptom could help define this time period as the Pre-SSc clinical phase although its specificity is low and its duration may be 5 years or more. Other parameters should be considered in the assessment of endothelial dysfunction, like capillaroscopic abnormalities, serum biomarkers (such as intercellular adhesion molecule-1, vascular cell adhesion molecule, anti-endothelial antibodies-1, or E-selectin or puffy fingers (PF)) [66]. In fact, puffy fingers have been proposed as an early sign of pre-scleroderma or VEDOSS and represent a continuum between these two entities and SSc [47]. Lescot suggested that PF may signify a vascular phenomenon such as is found in lcSSc or an early inflammatory phenomenon leading to dcSSc.

4.6 From ACR 1980 to VEDOSS criteria

In this gray area, in which the defined colors of the disease are still absent, and it is not yet possible to draw the patient's future, a very early diagnosis in a pre-clinical disease phase, and timely treatments, is the cornerstone for preventing disease evolution. If we review the road traveled by rheumatologists to achieve early diagnosis in SSc, we can see its beginnings in 1991 with the introduction of the term "early SSc" by Steen and Medsger [67]. They identified disease stages preceding the development of irreversible vascular damage and atrophic lesions in patients with definite diffuse

(<3 years from the first non-RP symptom) or limited SSc (<5 years), then also focusing on a temporal concept (number of years since the diagnosis).

In 1996, the term "pre-scleroderma" was proposed for the first time by Fine LG et al., and it identified patients with RP, digital ischemic abnormalities, and nailfold capillaroscopy findings (NFC) abnormalities or disease-specific circulating autoantibodies (i.e., anti-topoisomerase antibody, anticentromere antibody, anti RNA polymerase 3, antifibrillarin, anti-Th/To, or anti-PM-Scl) [60]. A few years later, a similar concept was named limited SSc (lSSc) by LeRoy and Medsger to describe patients with RP and either SSc-specific autoantibodies or SSc-type NFC pattern [61]. No other symptom/sign/laboratory findings were mentioned as necessary for the earliest diagnosis of SSc. Some patients with lSSc and without skin involvement, but with SSc NFC abnormalities, disease-specific antibodies, and/or internal organ involvement were called "SSc sine scleroderma" even if none of the registries published thus far have considered it [43]. Recently, Valentini et al. proposed the term "Undifferentiated Connective Tissue Disease at risk for Systemic Sclerosis" (UCTD-risk-SSc), to define a condition characterized by RP and either SSc-specific autoantibodies or a capillaroscopic scleroderma pattern or both, but without satisfying classification criteria for SSc, and also without features consistent with SSc sine scleroderma [68].

Two of the most important stages of this road toward defining an early diagnosis were the identification of the aforementioned "red flags," through a Delphi consensus study conducted by the European League Against Rheumatism (EULAR) Scleroderma Trial and Research (EUSTAR) among SSc experts. The consensus study proposed criteria for very early diagnosis of SSc (VEDOSS) [49] in 2011. This was followed by the publication of new ACR/EULAR classification criteria in 2013, in which the score of 9 was considered valid for classifying patients as SSc. This new definition allowed SSc-specific antibodies (ACA, ATA, and anti-RNA polymerase 3), capillaroscopy alterations (early signs of SSc), and more advanced features such as skin involvement, pulmonary involvement, and digital lesions.

The VEDOSS criteria defined ANA positivity, RP and PF as signs which should raise suspicion for SSc; if these were positive, it was suggested to examine SSc-specific antibodies (anticentromere, anti-topoisomerase (Scl-70), or anti-polymerase 3) and capillaroscopy. These criteria were validated in 2021 by a multicenter study that investigated the VEDOSS criteria to detect progression to classification criteria for SSc. This study evaluated 553 RP patients meeting the 5 VEDOSS criteria but not SSc criteria. At 5 years, 254 of the 553 (52.4%) were classified as EULAR/ACR 2013 SSc (**Table 2**). The study also reported that the absence of ANA decreased the risk of progression to SSc, (5-year progression 10–8%), while ANA positivity together with the presence of PF showed the highest rate of progression to 2013 ACR/EULARSSc criteria (79%). Particularly, ANA-positive patients with RP, SSc-specific autoantibodies, and PF had the highest progression rate over time (94.1%), followed by patients with ANA positive, specific autoantibodies, and NVC abnormalities (82.2%).

In clinical practice, when defining VEDOSS, several issues need to be addressed

1. "How many and which individual aspects of VEDOSS predict specific visceral involvement in SSc?

2. When should immunosuppressive treatment be started in VEDOSS?

3. Can starting vasoactive treatment very early prevent/delay the onset of pulmonary arterial hypertension or other vascular complications such as digital ulcers?

	Censored before 5 years (n = 299)	Five-year follow-up completers (n = 254)	P value	Total (n = 553)
Male	29 (9.7%)	17 (6.7%)	0.22	46 (8.3%)
Female	270 (90.3%)	237 (93.3%)	237 (93.3%)	507 (91.7%)
Age	43.63 (14.4)	48.7 (15.2)	<0.001	45.9 (15.0)
Duration of Raynaud's phenomenon (years)	4.0 (1.7–10.0)	4.0 (1.5–10.3)	0.98	4.0 (1.7–10.0)
ANA positive	187/293 (63.8%)	214/251 (85.3%)	<0.001	401/544 (73.7%)
Systemic sclerosis-specific autoantibody positive	77/280 (27.5%)	131/247 (53.0%)	<0.001	208/527 (39.5%)
Anticentromere antibody positive	64/275 (23.3%)	100/244 (41.0%)	<0.001	164/519 (31.6%)
Anti-scleroderma-70 positive	11/280 (3.9%)	28/245 (11.4%)	<0.001	39/525 (7.4%)
Anti-RNA polymerase III positive	2/109 (1.8%)	4/71 (5.6%)	0.21	6/180 (3.3%)
Puffy fingers	48/298 (16.1%)	48/242 (19.8%)	0.31	96/540 (17.8%)
Nailfold capillaroscopy abnormalities	105/286 (36.7%)	77/219 (35.2%)	0.78	182/505 (36.0%)

Table 2.
Characteristics of patients in the VEDOSS project [48].

4. Can we define what is the most appropriate follow-up timing in VEDOSS patients to avoid stressing patients without organ involvement?

5. Can other tests be useful for diagnosing VEDOSS or to define progression (e.g., lung ultrasound)?

6. Can hydroxychloroquine be useful to prevent progression?

These questions, and no doubt others, await research, assuming the acceptance of a uniform very early scleroderma definition (e.g., VEDOSS and SSc sine scleroderma).

5. Intrinsic gene subsets influence treatment response

The use of molecular phenotyping in SSc patients holds promise for guiding therapeutic approaches by tailoring treatments based on the individual's unique intrinsic gene subsets.

For example, it has been observed that SSc patients in the fibroproliferative gene subset tend to respond positively to tyrosine kinase inhibitors (TKIs), such as imatinib and nilotinib, which target tyrosine kinases involved in fibrotic pathways and reduced the expression of genes associated with the fibroproliferative subset in dcSSc patients. Similarly, higher baseline expression of genes related to TGFbR and PDGFR signaling in SSc patients correlated with positive responses to nilotinib. More recent trials analyzing the response to dasatinib also revealed that patients who showed improvement were predominantly from the fibroproliferative or normal-like subsets, while those who did not respond well were mainly from the inflammatory subsets [69–71].

Janus kinase (JAK), which is involved in cytokine signaling, has been implicated in the pathogenesis of SSc. Pre-clinical studies suggested its role in transmitting pro-inflammatory or profibrotic signals to target cells. Gene expression profiling analysis has confirmed elevated IL6/JAK/STAT gene signatures in skin biopsies of dcSSc patients belonging to the inflammatory subset, compared to healthy individuals.

The preliminary efficacy of tofacitinib, primarily an inhibitor of JAK1/3, was seen in the treatment of dcSSc patients with refractory skin involvement. A pilot study conducted at a single center evaluated the use of tofacitinib in a case series of 10 patients. The results showed a significant improvement in modified Rodnan skin score (mRSS) within the first month, indicating its potential as an effective immunosuppressant for progressive skin thickness in dcSSc [72]. Ongoing Phase I/II randomized controlled trials (NCT03274076) by Khanna et al. have shown initial results indicating the safety of tofacitinib and a trend toward mRSS improvement. Further studies are necessary to confirm the efficacy of tofacitinib and evaluate its response in relation to inflammatory and fibrotic gene signatures [73].

TGFb signaling targeted treatment (Fresolimumab) demonstrated efficacy in patients with high baseline levels of the TGFb-regulated gene thrombospondin-1 (THBS1). In those patients, THBS1 levels declined along with improved skin scores [74]. Taroni et al. conducted a functional genomic meta-analysis, using publicly available gene expression data from clinical trials of various therapeutics including MMF and fresolimumab. The analysis revealed that improvers on fresolimumab had high baseline levels of TGFb-related genes, while non-improvers had elevated levels of immune-related genes at baseline. Conversely, MMF improvers had high baseline levels of immune-related genes that decreased after treatment [59]. This study emphasizes the importance of genome-wide gene expression data collected during clinical trials.

Patients who responded to immunosuppressive medications were more likely to be associated with inflammatory gene subsets. For instance, responders to mycophenolate mofetil (MMF), which targets lymphocyte proliferation, belonged to the inflammatory gene subset (four out of seven improvers), while non-improvers were associated with the fibroproliferative gene subset (two subjects) [75]. Similarly, responders to abatacept, which inhibits CD28 T-cell activation, had positive responses among patients in the inflammatory gene subset. Improvers who responded to abatacept (four out of five), were primarily associated with the inflammatory gene subset and had higher baseline levels of CD28 signaling. On the other hand, the non-improver (one patient) belonged to the normal-like gene subset and exhibited lower baseline levels of CD28 signaling [76].

In summary, these findings demonstrate the relevance of intrinsic gene subsets and their relationship with specific treatment responses. They emphasize the potential for using genomic data to inform treatment decisions and personalize therapeutic approaches in SSc patients.

6. Classification according to abnormal nailfold capillaroscopy findings (NFC) patterns

Abnormal NFC can be classified as early, active, or late, providing valuable insights into the overall progression of the disease. The severity of NFC patterns has been identified as a predictive factor for future severe organ involvement, although it requires years to manifest. This slowly changing risk tends to increase as the NFC pattern progresses from early to late, even after accounting for disease duration, subset, and vasoactive medications [49, 77–79].

NFC and laboratory tools (gene signatures and autoantibodies) into a classification system have the potential to develop a more comprehensive and predictive approach. This integration can inform treatment decisions and ultimately lead to improved personalized/precision patient outcomes [80].

7. Conclusion

While the classification criteria for SSc have been carefully delineated, the definition of what comes before meeting classification criteria is not so well understood. For systemic sclerosis, there may well be a very early SSc phase before any but constitutional symptoms occur, associated with varying degrees of genetic and serological signals. The very early diagnosis of systemic sclerosis (VEDOSS) has been defined and is useful. However, there remain multiple questions surrounding VEDOSS, including when and how to treat patients with this diagnosis.

The identification of validated biomarkers and genetic predictors for disease susceptibility and progression would allow risk stratification of patients and subsequent tailored clinical and therapeutic management and an efficient use of resources. However, despite progress, there are as yet no fully validated biomarkers or genetic predictors for disease evolution.

Proportion fulfilling 2013 ACR-EULAR criteria		**ANA**	**Ssc-Ab**	**SSc pattern on NFC**	**Puffy fingers**
In the presence of	ANA	58.9%	70.2%	75.0%	79.0%
	SSc-Ab	70.2%	70.2%	82.2%	94.1%
	SSc pattern on NVC	75.0%	82.2%	70.1%	69.2%
	Puffy fingers	79.0%	94.1%	69.2%	70.8%
In the absence of	ANA	10.8%	31.0%	40.4%	47.5%
	SSc-Ab	31.0%	31.0%	41.9%	49.6%
	SSc pattern on NFC	40.4%	41.9%	41.5%	50.9%
	Puffy fingers	47.5%	49.6%	50.9%	47.9%

Table 3.
Frequency of progression as calculated in the presence or absence of the VEDOSS criteria alone or in combination [47–49].

Moreover, although VEDOSS patients with RP, autoantibodies, and SSc capillaroscopic pattern could be followed up, we have not yet developed a cohort study, documenting all appropriate clinical, genetic, and autoimmune measures, followed for at least 5 and perhaps more years, using a randomized menu of treatments (**Table 3**).

Acknowledgements

I wish to acknowledge the diligent and ongoing work of Claudia Real, my executive assistant, without whom this chapter would never have been completed.

Disclosures

Bellando-Randone S.—none declared; Suliman Y.—none declared; Anwar S.—none declared; Furst D.E.—none declared.

Author details

Silvia Bellando-Randone[1], Yossra Suliman[2], Sana Anwar[3] and Daniel E. Furst[1,4,5]*

1 University of Florence, Florence, Italy

2 Assiut University, Assuit, Egypt

3 Lugansk State Medical University, Ukraine

4 University of California in Los Angeles, USA

5 University of Washington, Seattle, Washington, USA

*Address all correspondence to: dan@furst.us.com

References

[1] Goetz LH, Schork NJ. Personalized medicine: Motivation, challenges, and progress. Fertility and Sterility. 2018;**109**(6):952-963

[2] Czirjak L, Matucci-Cerinic M. Beyond Raynaud's phenomenon hides very early systemic sclerosis: The assessment of organ involvement is always mandatory. Rheumatology (Oxford, England). 2011;**50**(2):250-251

[3] Haque A, Hughes M. Raynaud's phenomenon. Clinical Medicine (London, England). 2020;**20**(6):580-587

[4] Romanowska-Prochnicka K, Walczyk M, Olesinska M. Recognizing systemic sclerosis: Comparative analysis of various sets of classification criteria. Reumatologia. 2016;**54**(6):296-305

[5] van den Hoogen F, Khanna D, Fransen J, Johnson SR, Baron M, Tyndall A, et al. 2013 classification criteria for systemic sclerosis: An American college of rheumatology/European league against rheumatism collaborative initiative. Annals of the Rheumatic Diseases. 2013;**72**(11):1747-1755

[6] Arend WP, Firestein GS. Pre-rheumatoid arthritis: Predisposition and transition to clinical synovitis. Nature Reviews Rheumatology. 2012;**8**(10):573-586

[7] Aletaha D, Neogi T, Silman AJ, Funovits J, Felson DT, Bingham CO 3rd, et al. 2010 Rheumatoid arthritis classification criteria: An American College of Rheumatology/European League Against Rheumatism collaborative initiative. Arthritis and Rheumatism. 2010;**62**(9):2569-2581

[8] Karlson EW, Deane K. Environmental and gene-environment interactions and risk of rheumatoid arthritis. Rheumatic Diseases Clinics of North America. 2012;**38**(2):405-426

[9] Padyukov L, Silva C, Stolt P, Alfredsson L, Klareskog L. A gene-environment interaction between smoking and shared epitope genes in HLA-DR provides a high risk of seropositive rheumatoid arthritis. Arthritis and Rheumatism. 2004;**50**(10):3085-3092

[10] Greenblatt HK, Kim HA, Bettner LF, Deane KD. Preclinical rheumatoid arthritis and rheumatoid arthritis prevention. Current Opinion in Rheumatology. 2020;**32**(3):289-296

[11] Sugiyama D, Nishimura K, Tamaki K, Tsuji G, Nakazawa T, Morinobu A, et al. Impact of smoking as a risk factor for developing rheumatoid arthritis: A meta-analysis of observational studies. Annals of the Rheumatic Diseases. 2010;**69**(1):70-81

[12] Gerlag DM, Raza K, van Baarsen LG, Brouwer E, Buckley CD, Burmester GR, et al. EULAR recommendations for terminology and research in individuals at risk of rheumatoid arthritis: Report from the Study Group for Risk Factors for Rheumatoid Arthritis. Annals of the Rheumatic Diseases. 2012;**71**(5):638-641

[13] van Steenbergen HW, Aletaha D, Beaart-van de Voorde LJ, Brouwer E, Codreanu C, Combe B, et al. EULAR definition of arthralgia suspicious for progression to rheumatoid arthritis. Annals of the Rheumatic Diseases. 2017;**76**(3):491-496

[14] Raza K, Gerlag DM. Preclinical inflammatory rheumatic diseases: An overview and relevant nomenclature.

Rheumatic Diseases Clinics of North America. 2014;**40**(4):569-580

[15] van Vollenhoven RF. Sex differences in rheumatoid arthritis: More than meets the eye. BMC Medicine. 2009;**7**:12

[16] Wellcome Trust Case Control Consortium. Genome-wide association study of 14,000 cases of seven common diseases and 3,000 shared controls. Nature. 2007;**447**(7145):661-678

[17] Costenbader KH, Feskanich D, Mandl LA, Karlson EW. Smoking intensity, duration, and cessation, and the risk of rheumatoid arthritis in women. The American Journal of Medicine. 2006;**119**(6):503.e1-503.e9

[18] Martinez-Martinez RE, Abud-Mendoza C, Patino-Marin N, Rizo-Rodriguez JC, Little JW, Loyola-Rodriguez JP. Detection of periodontal bacterial DNA in serum and synovial fluid in refractory rheumatoid arthritis patients. Journal of Clinical Periodontology. 2009;**36**(12):1004-1010

[19] Li S, Yu Y, Yue Y, Zhang Z, Su K. Microbial infection and rheumatoid arthritis. Journal of Clinical and Cellular Immunology. 2013;**4**(6):174. DOI: 10.4174/2155-9899.190174

[20] Fechtner S, Berens H, Bemis E, Johnson RL, Guthridge CJ, Carlson NE, et al. Antibody responses to Epstein-Barr virus in the preclinical period of rheumatoid arthritis suggest the presence of increased viral reactivation cycles. Arthritis & Rhematology. 2022;**74**(4):597-603

[21] Feng X, Xu X, Shi Y, Liu X, Liu H, Hou H, et al. Body mass index and the risk of rheumatoid arthritis: An updated dose-response meta-analysis. BioMed Research International. 2019;**2019**:3579081

[22] Romão VC, Fonseca JE. Etiology and risk factors for rheumatoid arthritis: A state-of-the-art review. Frontiers in Medicine (Lausanne) 2021;**8**:689698. DOI: 10.3389/fmed.2021.689698. PMID: 34901047; PMCID: PMC8661097

[23] Lei Y, Li X, Gao Z, Liu Y, Zhang B, Xia L, et al. Association between adiponectin and clinical manifestations in rheumatoid arthritis. Journal of Interferon & Cytokine Research. 2020;**40**(10):501-508

[24] Alpizar-Rodriguez D, Pluchino N, Canny G, Gabay C, Finckh A. The role of female hormonal factors in the development of rheumatoid arthritis. Rheumatology (Oxford, England). 2017;**56**(8):1254-1263

[25] Kremer JM. n-3 fatty acid supplements in rheumatoid arthritis. The American Journal of Clinical Nutrition. 2000;**71**(Suppl. 1):349S-351S

[26] Gioia C, Lucchino B, Tarsitano MG, Iannuccelli C, Di Franco M. Dietary habits and nutrition in rheumatoid arthritis: Can diet influence disease development and clinical manifestations? Nutrients. 2020;**12**(5):1456. DOI: 103390/NU12051456

[27] Ingegnoli F, Castelli R, Gualtierotti R. Rheumatoid factors: Clinical applications. Disease Markers. 2013;**35**(6):727-734

[28] Nielen MM, van Schaardenburg D, Reesink HW, van de Stadt RJ, van der Horst-Bruinsma IE, de Koning MH, et al. Specific autoantibodies precede the symptoms of rheumatoid arthritis: A study of serial measurements in blood donors. Arthritis and Rheumatism. 2004;**50**(2):380-386

[29] Kurowska W, Kuca-Warnawin EH, Radzikowska A, Maslinski W. The

role of anti-citrullinated protein antibodies (ACPA) in the pathogenesis of rheumatoid arthritis. Central European Journal of Immunology. 2017;**42**(4):390-398

[30] Aggarwal R, Liao K, Nair R, Ringold S, Costenbader KH. Anti-citrullinated peptide antibody assays and their role in the diagnosis of rheumatoid arthritis. Arthritis and Rheumatism. 2009;**61**(11):1472-1483

[31] Mun S, Lee J, Park M, Shin J, Lim MK, Kang HG. Serum biomarker panel for the diagnosis of rheumatoid arthritis. Arthritis Research & Therapy. 2021;**23**(1):31

[32] Deane KD, Holers VM. Rheumatoid arthritis pathogenesis, prediction, and prevention: An emerging paradigm shift. Arthritis & Rhematology. 2021;**73**(2):181-193

[33] Turk SA, van Beers-Tas MH, van Schaardenburg D. Prediction of future rheumatoid arthritis. Rheumatic Diseases Clinics of North America. 2014;**40**(4):753-770

[34] Emery P, Gabay C, Kraan M, Gomez-Reino J. Evidence-based review of biologic markers as indicators of disease progression and remission in rheumatoid arthritis. Rheumatology International. 2007;**27**(9):793-806

[35] Shapiro SC. Biomarkers in rheumatoid arthritis. Cureus. 2021;**13**(5):e15063

[36] Ricchiuti V, Chun KY, Yang JM, Aure MA, Gomez L, Norman GL, et al. Anti-carbamylated protein (anti-CarP) antibodies in patients evaluated for suspected rheumatoid arthritis. Diagnostics (Basel). 2022;**12**(7):1661-1670

[37] Li L, Deng C, Chen S, Zhang S, Wu Z, Hu C, et al. Meta-analysis: Diagnostic accuracy of anti-carbamylated protein antibody for rheumatoid arthritis. PLoS ONE. 2016;**11**(7):e0159000

[38] Bergstedt DT, Tarter WJ, Peterson RA, Feser ML, Parish MC, Striebich CC, et al. Antibodies to citrullinated protein antigens, rheumatoid factor isotypes and the shared epitope and the near-term development of clinically-apparent rheumatoid arthritis. Frontiers in Immunology. 2022;**13**:916277

[39] Wysocki T, Olesinska M, Paradowska-Gorycka A. Current understanding of an emerging role of HLA-DRB1 gene in rheumatoid arthritis-from research to clinical practice. Cells. 2020;**9**(5):1127-1143

[40] Gerlag DM, Safy M, Maijer KI, Tang MW, Tas SW, Starmans-Kool MJF, et al. Effects of B-cell directed therapy on the preclinical stage of rheumatoid arthritis: The PRAIRI study. Annals of the Rheumatic Diseases. 2019;**78**(2):179-185

[41] Burgers LE, Allaart CF, Huizinga TWJ, van der Helm-van Mil AHM. Brief report: Clinical trials aiming to prevent rheumatoid arthritis cannot detect prevention without adequate risk stratification: A trial of methotrexate versus placebo in undifferentiated arthritis as an example. Arthritis & Rhematology. 2017;**69**(5):926-931

[42] Emery P, Durez P, Dougados M, Legerton CW, Becker JC, Vratsanos G, et al. Impact of T-cell costimulation modulation in patients with undifferentiated inflammatory arthritis or very early rheumatoid arthritis: A clinical and imaging study of abatacept (the ADJUST trial). Annals of the Rheumatic Diseases. 2010;**69**(3):510-516

[43] Bellando-Randone S, Matucci-Cerinic M. Very early systemic sclerosis. Best Practice & Research. Clinical Rheumatology. 2019;**33**(4):101428

[44] Minier T, Pentek M, Brodszky V, Ecseki A, Karpati K, Polgar A, et al. Cost-of-illness of patients with systemic sclerosis in a tertiary care Centre. Rheumatology (Oxford, England). 2010;**49**(10):1920-1928

[45] Elhai M, Meune C, Avouac J, Kahan A, Allanore Y. Trends in mortality in patients with systemic sclerosis over 40 years: A systematic review and meta-analysis of cohort studies. Rheumatology (Oxford, England). 2012;**51**(6):1017-1026

[46] Jaafar S, Lescoat A, Huang S, Gordon J, Hinchcliff M, Shah AA, et al. Clinical characteristics, visceral involvement, and mortality in at-risk or early diffuse systemic sclerosis: A longitudinal analysis of an observational prospective multicenter US cohort. Arthritis Research & Therapy. 2021;**23**(1):170

[47] Lescoat A. Very early diagnosis of systemic sclerosis: Deciphering the heterogeneity of systemic sclerosis in the very early stages of the disease. Journal of Scleroderma and Related Disorders. 2023;**8**(1):3-6

[48] Bellando-Randone S. Progression of patients with Raynaud's phenomenon to systemic sclerosis: A five-year analysis of the European Scleroderma Trial and Research group multicentre, longitudinal registry study for Very Early Diagnosis of Systemic Sclerosis. The Lancet Rheumatology. 2021;**3**(12):e834-ee43

[49] Avouac J, Fransen J, Walker UA, Riccieri V, Smith V, Muller C, et al. Preliminary criteria for the very early diagnosis of systemic sclerosis: Results of a Delphi Consensus Study from EULAR Scleroderma Trials and Research Group. Annals of the Rheumatic Diseases. 2011;**70**(3):476-481

[50] Nihtyanova SI, Denton CP. Autoantibodies as predictive tools in systemic sclerosis. Nature Reviews Rheumatology. 2010;**6**(2):112-116

[51] Boonstra M, Mertens BJA, Bakker JA, Ninaber MK, Marsan NA, van der Helm-van Mil, AHM, et al. To what extent do autoantibodies help to identify high-risk patients in systemic sclerosis? Clinical and Experimental Rheumatology. 2018;(Suppl 113):109-117

[52] Sobanski V, Giovannelli J, Allanore Y, Riemekasten G, Airo P, Vettori S, et al. Phenotypes determined by cluster analysis and their survival in the prospective European scleroderma trials and research cohort of patients with systemic sclerosis. Arthritis & Rhematology. 2019;**71**(9):1553-1570

[53] van der Kroef M, van den Hoogen LL, Mertens JS, Blokland SLM, Haskett S, Devaprasad A, et al. Cytometry by time of flight identifies distinct signatures in patients with systemic sclerosis, systemic lupus erythematosus and Sjogrens syndrome. European Journal of Immunology. 2020;**50**(1):119-129

[54] Makinde HM, Dunn JLM, Gadhvi G, Carns M, Aren K, Chung AH, et al. Three distinct transcriptional profiles of monocytes associate with disease activity in scleroderma patients. Arthritis & Rhematology. 2023;**75**(4):595-608

[55] Pendergrass SA, Lemaire R, Francis IP, Mahoney JM, Lafyatis R, Whitfield ML. Intrinsic gene expression subsets of diffuse cutaneous systemic sclerosis are stable in serial skin biopsies. The Journal of Investigative Dermatology. 2012;**132**(5):1363-1373

[56] Milano A, Pendergrass SA, Sargent JL, George LK, McCalmont TH,

Connolly MK, et al. Molecular subsets in the gene expression signatures of scleroderma skin. PLoS ONE. 2008;**3**(7):e2696

[57] Skaug B, Lyons MA, Swindell WR, Salazar GA, Wu M, Tran TM, et al. Large-scale analysis of longitudinal skin gene expression in systemic sclerosis reveals relationships of immune cell and fibroblast activity with skin thickness and a trend towards normalisation over time. Annals of the Rheumatic Diseases. 2022;**81**(4):516-523

[58] Taroni JN, Martyanov V, Huang CC, Mahoney JM, Hirano I, Shetuni B, et al. Molecular characterization of systemic sclerosis esophageal pathology identifies inflammatory and proliferative signatures. Arthritis Research & Therapy. 2015;**17**:194

[59] Taroni JN, Martyanov V, Mahoney JM, Whitfield ML. A functional genomic meta-analysis of clinical trials in systemic sclerosis: Toward precision medicine and combination therapy. The Journal of Investigative Dermatology. 2017;**137**(5):1033-1041

[60] No Authors. Systemic sclerosis: Current pathogenetic concepts and future prospects for targeted therapy. Lancet. 1996;**347**(9013):1453-1458

[61] LeRoy EC, Medsger TA Jr. Criteria for the classification of early systemic sclerosis. The Journal of Rheumatology. 2001;**28**(7):1573-1576

[62] Pope JE, Al-Bishri J, Al-Azem H, Ouimet JM. The temporal relationship of Raynaud's phenomenon and features of connective tissue disease in rheumatoid arthritis. The Journal of Rheumatology. 2008;**35**(12):2329-2333

[63] Mosca M, Tani C, Talarico R, Bombardieri S. Undifferentiated connective tissue diseases (UCTD): Simplified systemic autoimmune diseases. Autoimmunity Reviews. 2011;**10**(5):256-258

[64] Gunnarsson R, Hetlevik SO, Lilleby V, Molberg O. Mixed connective tissue disease. Best Practice & Research. Clinical Rheumatology. 2016;**30**(1):95-111

[65] Meier FM, Frommer KW, Dinser R, Walker UA, Czirjak L, Denton CP, et al. Update on the profile of the EUSTAR cohort: An analysis of the EULAR Scleroderma Trials and Research group database. Annals of the Rheumatic Diseases. 2012;**71**(8):1355-1360

[66] Denton CP, Bickerstaff MC, Shiwen X, Carulli MT, Haskard DO, Dubois RM, et al. Serial circulating adhesion molecule levels reflect disease severity in systemic sclerosis. British Journal of Rheumatology. 1995;**34**(11):1048-1054

[67] Steen VD, Medsger TA Jr. Epidemiology and natural history of systemic sclerosis. Rheumatic Diseases Clinics of North America. 1990;**16**(1):1-10

[68] Valentini G. Undifferentiated Connective Tissue Disease at risk for systemic sclerosis (SSc) (so far referred to as very early/early SSc or pre-SSc). Autoimmunity Reviews. 2015;**14**(3):210-213

[69] Chung L, Fiorentino DF, Benbarak MJ, Adler AS, Mariano MM, Paniagua RT, et al. Molecular framework for response to imatinib mesylate in systemic sclerosis. Arthritis and Rheumatism. 2009;**60**(2):584-591

[70] Gordon JK, Martyanov V, Magro C, Wildman HF, Wood TA, Huang WT, et al. Nilotinib (Tasigna) in the treatment

of early diffuse systemic sclerosis: An open-label, pilot clinical trial. Arthritis Research & Therapy. 2015;**17**(1):213

[71] Martyanov V, Kim GJ, Hayes W, Du S, Ganguly BJ, Sy O, et al. Novel lung imaging biomarkers and skin gene expression subsetting in dasatinib treatment of systemic sclerosis-associated interstitial lung disease. PLoS ONE. 2017;**12**(11):e0187580

[72] You H, Xu D, Hou Y, Zhou J, Wang Q, Li M, et al. Tofacitinib as a possible treatment for skin thickening in diffuse cutaneous systemic sclerosis. Rheumatology (Oxford, England). 2021;**60**(5):2472-2477

[73] Khanna DBE, Nagaraja V, Koenig A, Khanna P, Young A, et al. Tofacitinib in early diffuse cutaneous systemic sclerosis-results of phase I/II investigator-initiated, double-blind randomized placebo-controlled trial. Arthritis and Rheumatology. 2019;**71**(11):1493-1495

[74] Rice LM, Padilla CM, McLaughlin SR, Mathes A, Ziemek J, Goummih S, et al. Fresolimumab treatment decreases biomarkers and improves clinical symptoms in systemic sclerosis patients. The Journal of Clinical Investigation. 2015;**125**(7):2795-2807

[75] Hinchcliff M, Huang CC, Wood TA, Matthew Mahoney J, Martyanov V, Bhattacharyya S, et al. Molecular signatures in skin associated with clinical improvement during mycophenolate treatment in systemic sclerosis. The Journal of Investigative Dermatology. 2013;**133**(8):1979-1989

[76] Chakravarty EF, Martyanov V, Fiorentino D, Wood TA, Haddon DJ, Jarrell JA, et al. Gene expression changes reflect clinical response in a placebo-controlled randomized trial of abatacept in patients with diffuse cutaneous systemic sclerosis. Arthritis Research & Therapy. 2015;**17**(1):159

[77] Ingegnoli F, Ardoino I, Boracchi P, Cutolo M, co-authors E. Nailfold capillaroscopy in systemic sclerosis: Data from the EULAR scleroderma trials and research (EUSTAR) database. Microvascular Research. 2013;**89**:122-128

[78] Smith V, Riccieri V, Pizzorni C, Decuman S, Deschepper E, Bonroy C, et al. Nailfold capillaroscopy for prediction of novel future severe organ involvement in systemic sclerosis. The Journal of Rheumatology. 2013;**40**(12):2023-2028

[79] Smith V, Decuman S, Sulli A, Bonroy C, Piettte Y, Deschepper E, et al. Do worsening scleroderma capillaroscopic patterns predict future severe organ involvement? A pilot study. Annals of the Rheumatic Diseases. 2012;**71**(10):1636-1639

[80] Noviani M, Chellamuthu VR, Albani S, Low AHL. Toward molecular stratification and precision medicine in systemic sclerosis. Frontiers in Medicine (Lausanne). 2022;**9**:911977

Chapter 4

Diagnostic Methods for Microvasculopathy in Systemic Sclerosis

Bartosz Miziołek, Michał Szczepanek and Beata Bergler-Czop

Abstract

A generalized damage to the microcirculation (microvasculopathy) is a cardinal feature of systemic sclerosis and its first manifestation is Raynaud's phenomenon. Early detection of microvasculopathy enables to establish the right diagnosis at the very early stage of the disease and to identify those patients with the greater risk of internal organ involvement or developmental digital tip ulcers. Dynamic methods help to monitor the response to treatment that influences on the vasomotoric functions of the microcirculation. The gold standard for the assessment of microvascular involvement constitutes nailfold capillaroscopy, which can be performed using stereomicroscopy, videocapillaroscopy, or dermoscopy. Other non-invasive diagnostic methods include sidestream dark field imaging, optical coherence tomography, laser Doppler and laser-related methods, and thermography.

Keywords: microvasculopathy, nailfold capillaroscopy, dermoscopy, sidestream dark field imaging laser methods, optical coherence tomography, doppler methods, thermography, systemic sclerosis

1. Introduction

A generalized damage to the microcirculation (microvasculopathy) is a cardinal feature of systemic sclerosis (SSc) and its first manifestation is Raynaud's phenomenon (RP) [1]. The gold standard for the assessment of microvascular involvement constitutes nailfold capillaroscopy (NFC), but attempts to evaluate the microcirculation in nailfolds date back to 1912. Warren Lombard from the Physiological Institute of the University of Würzburg found improved visibility of dermal papillae and the superficial blood vessels after application of glycerine and transparent oil on the skin [2]. This proposal to use immersion oils for visual exploration of skin capillaries allowed for later development of nailfold capillaroscopic assessment in patients with scleroderma by Brown and O'Leary with stereomicroscope [3]. Intense works of Maricq's and LeRoy brought the renaissance on the use of NFC in the diagnostic management of systemic sclerosis [4–6].

2. Nailfold capillaroscopy (NFC)

NFC is the first step at the diagnostic management in patients with RP to distinguish primary from secondary symptom. Abnormalities seen in NFC in patients with RP which coexist with positivity to specific for SSc antinuclear antibodies help to identify those subjects at the very early stage of the disease [7]. SSc is the only systemic connective tissue disease (CTD), which includes capillaroscopic abnormalities in classification criteria established by the European League Against Rheumatism and American College of Rheumatology [8]. The significance of NFC for other CTDs is lower and neither classification criteria for systemic lupus erythematosus [9] nor ones for idiopathic inflammatory myopathies [10] require evaluation of nailfolds. NFC does not only help to establish the diagnosis of SSc, but it also enables to follow-up a progression of microvasculopathy [11]. Capillaroscopic patterns proposed more than twenty years ago by Cutolo et al. (**Figure 1**) have been still the most valuable grading tool for the damage to the microcirculation [12].

Although microvasculopathy in SSc is generalized, the damage to the microcirculation is preferentially evaluated in nailfolds of fingers. Skin capillaries are parallel to the epidermis in nailfolds, while in other areas of the body they run perpendicularly (**Figure 2**). This parallel arrangement allows the observation of the capillaries along instead of only their top-like features in the majority of body surface [13, 14]. One may notice there is an easy development of multiple telangiectasia in patients with SSc due to a ramification of microvessels, which run parallel to the epidermis. Their shape and arrangement are mostly randomized and less predictable than in nailfolds, as well as these telangiectasias may overlap with physiologically already developed ones [15]. Overall, the standardization for the assessment of microvasculopathy in patients with Raynaud's phenomenon and systemic sclerosis was developed by the European Scleroderma Trials and Research group only in fingers [1].

Initially enlarged capillary loops and then megacapillaries, cap hemorrhages, bushy, and ramified vascular loops, together with disarrangement of vascularity and avascular areas, are typically seen in nailfolds of patients with SSc (**Figure 3**) [12]. The microcirculation in nailfolds can be evaluated with a use of stereomicroscope, USB microscope (including a dedicated videocapillaroscope), as well as handheld dermoscope.

Stereomicroscopy (**Figure 4**) helped to develop NFC technique yet by Brown and O'Leary [3] or later by Maricq and LeRoy [4–6]. It shows capillaries at 10–40

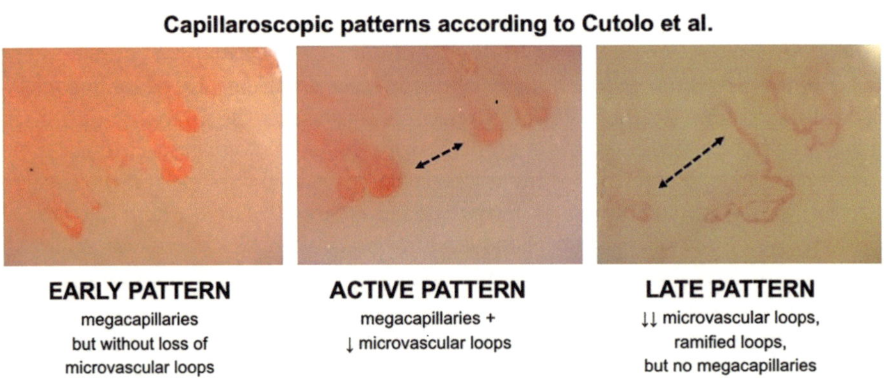

Figure 1.
Classification of microvasculopathy to capillaroscopic patterns.

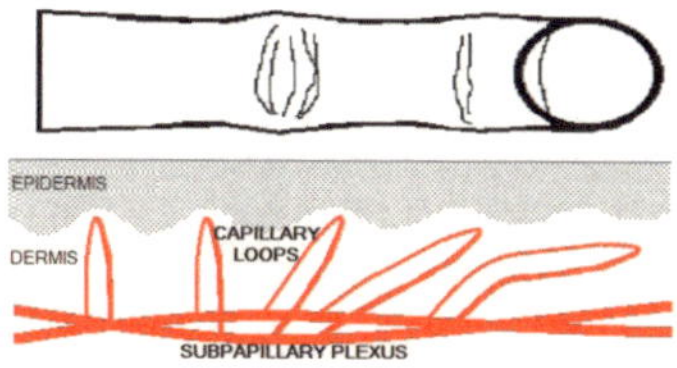

Figure 2.
Capillary loops in the papillary dermis run mostly perpendicularly but in nailfolds they are distributed parallelly to the epidermis.

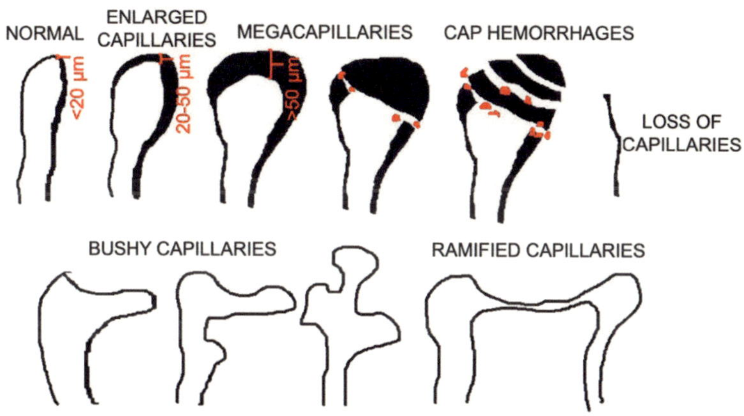

Figure 3.
Different forms of capillary loops seen typically in patients with systemic sclerosis with the possibility of measuring diameter of capillary loop at the apical part of the vascular loop.

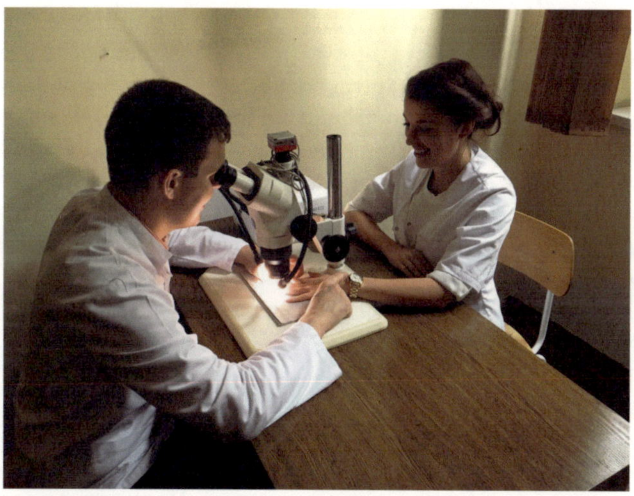

Figure 4.
NFC with the use of stereomicroscopy.

magnification, which allows for widefield evaluation of capillary loops in the entire nailfold; however, stereomicroscopy shares same limitations. Firstly, it is non-portable technique, which requires an additional lighting with a fiber-optic illuminator.

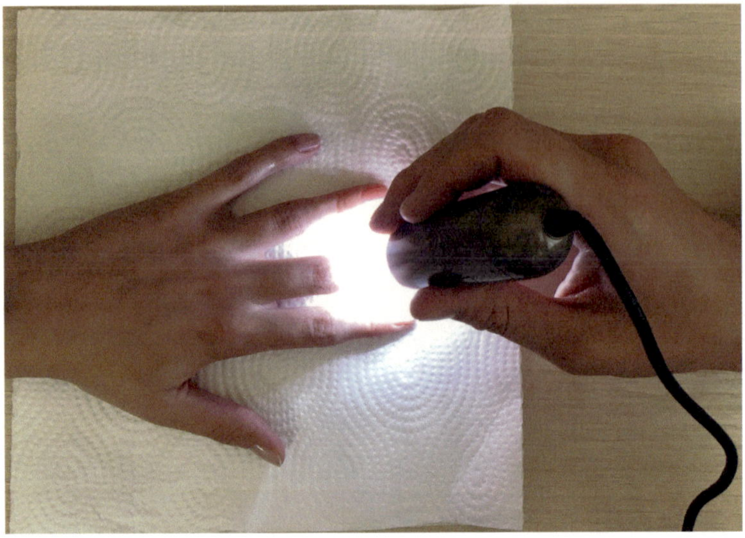

Figure 5.
NFC with use of nailfold videocapillaroscopy.

The distance between the optical system of the stereomicroscope and the nailfold may require additional fixation of the finger to capture sharp pictures of capillaries. Space restriction between the objective and the stage may limit the use of stereomicroscopy in case of flexural contracture of fingers developing in some of SSc patients.

Development of USB microscopy has enabled to perform NFC at the bed of patient even in case of advanced deformation of fingers. Dedicated videocapillaroscopy systems (**Figure 5**) may show vascular loops with 50–600 magnification and they are equipped with integrated LED diodes that illuminate the nailfold. High-power magnification restricts, however, the assessment of the nailfold to only selected region at a time in a contrast to stereomicroscopy, which allows for a quick global evaluation of the microcirculation in the nailfold due to the widefield of vision. Direct contact with the finger shortens the distance between the optical axis and the nailfold, which reduces the blur of pictures due to the movements of fingers. Capillaries are mostly sharply visible on pictures, which enable for their further qualitative and quantitative assessment with the use of dedicated software systems [16, 17].

3. Dermoscopy

Dermoscopy is an imagining technique primarily used by dermatologists for evaluation of pigmental lesions, but it was shown to be sufficient for early assessment of microvessels. A handheld device reveals vascular structures at the nailfold with a standard 10-fold magnification (**Figures 6–8**), which may help to distinguish normal from abnormal microcirculation at the first consultation of a patient with RP. Identification of abnormalities of microvessels usually requires referring the patient to a full NFC at greater magnification for detailed analysis of nailfolds. Attachment of dermoscope to a smartphone may enhance the magnification increasing the zoom up to 20–30× (**Figures 9–11**), therefore allowing for more precise evaluation of the

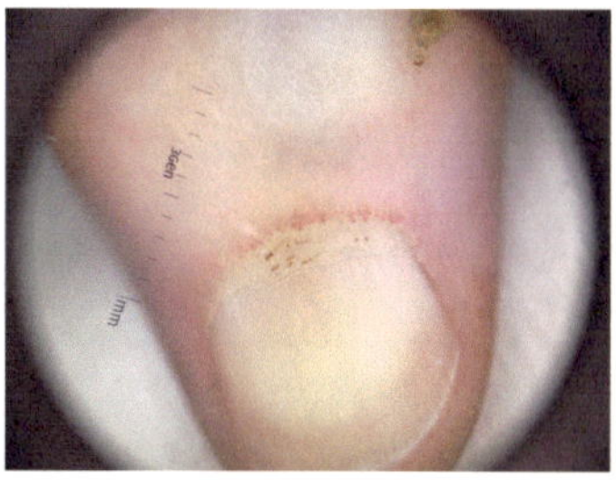

Figure 6.
NFC with the use of dermoscopy (10× zoom).

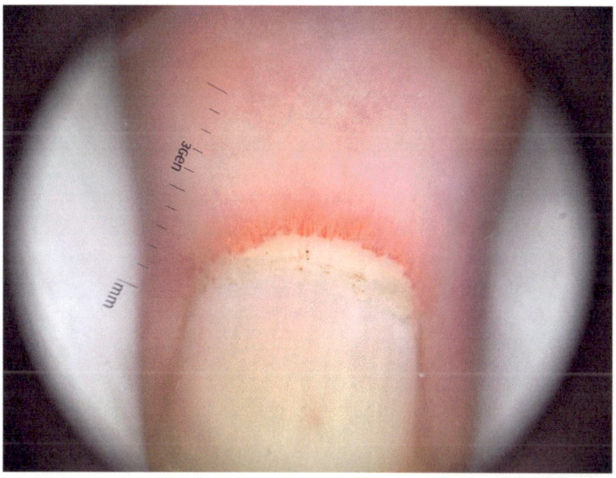

Figure 7.
Megacapillaries seen under dermoscopy in nailfolds (10× zoom).

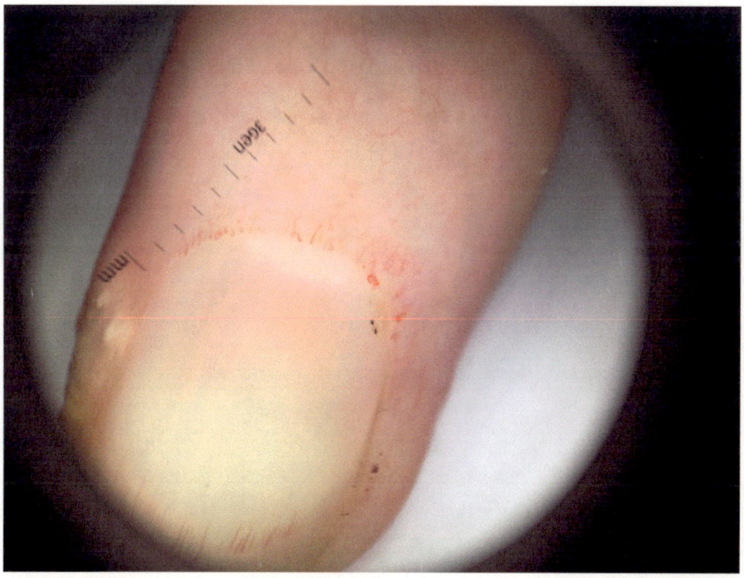

Figure 8.
Megacapillaries and microaneurysma seen under dermoscopy in nailfolds (10× zoom).

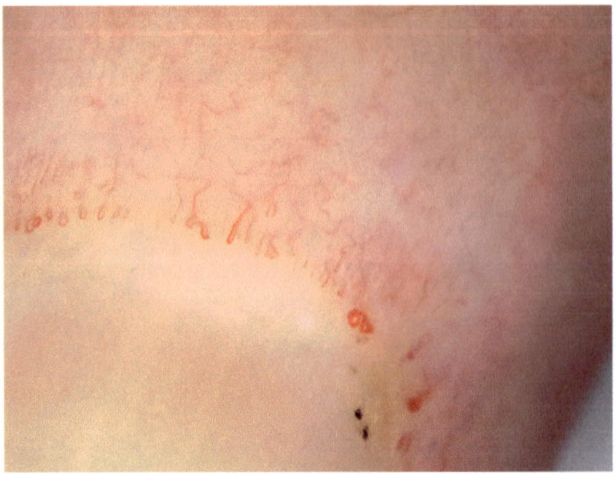

Figure 9.
Megacapillaries, microaneurysma and ramified capillaries seen under dermoscopy in nailfolds (20× zoom enhanced by smartphone).

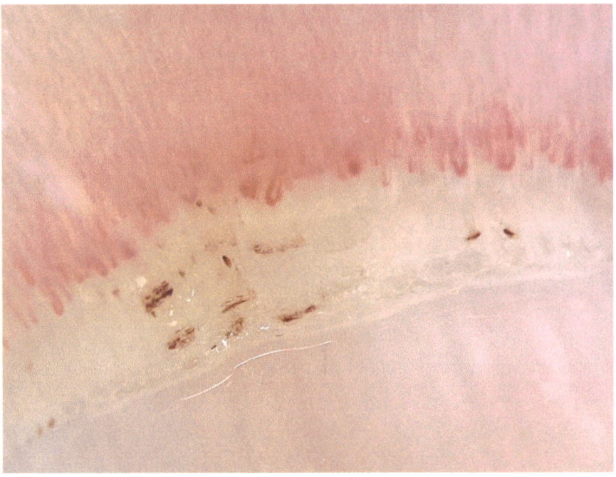

Figure 10.
NFC with the use of dermoscopy after attachment to smartphone (20× zoom).

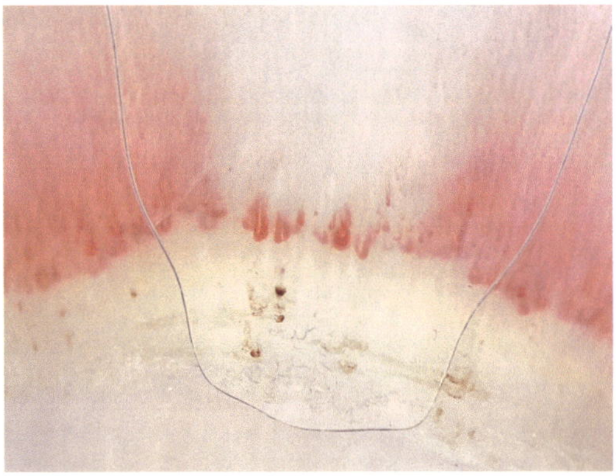

Figure 11.
Pseudo-avascularization due to the squeezing of microvessels by dermoscope (20× zoom enhanced by smartphone).

microcirculation and its classification to capillaroscopic patterns [18]. One should remember not to lean the dermoscope firmly on the nailfold to avoid squeezing the vessels and the appearance of pseudo-avascularization (**Figure 11**).

4. Sidestream dark field imaging

The generalized microvasculopathy contributes to the involvement of other than cutaneous vascular bed. There was proposed evaluation of the microcirculation in oral cavity by sidestream dark field imaging, which is an automatic real-time microcirculation analysis tool. Evaluation of the capillary bed in the sublingual region showed previously significantly lower capillary density in SSc patients than in healthy controls [19, 20]. There were found positive correlations between NFC and sublingual measurement of perfusion and capillary density [20].

5. Optical coherence tomography

The involvement of the microcirculation in the eye was investigated using optical coherence tomography angiography (OCTA). It showed significantly reduced both retinal and choroidal perfusions in SSc patients when compared to controls [21, 22]. The use of optical coherence tomography of the skin showed earlier to be a valuable assessment tool potent to obtain virtual skin biopsy. A use of infrared light enables to produce images of micron resolution. OCT A-scans were previously referred to skin biopsies obtained in SSc patients from fingers (dorsal and volar aspect), hand (dorsal aspect), and forearm (dorsal and volar aspect). These images revealed blurred dermal-epidermal junction and the loss of capillaries in the skin of SSc patients [23]. A flow in the cutaneous microcirculation can be better explored with newly developed dynamic OCT (D-OCT). It recently demonstrated the reduced blood flow in nailfolds according to capillaroscopic patterns, but only a moderate correlation was seen between microvascular flow density measured by D-OCT and the number of capillaries calculated in NFC. One should notice that D-OCT analyzes the blood perfusion in a portion of the skin (3D space), whereas NFC counts capillaries only in the distal raw of the nailfold (2D surface) [24].

6. Laser doppler and laser related methods

A measurement of a shift in light beam backscattered by moving erythrocytes is the basis of laser Doppler techniques (**Figure 12**). Laser Doppler flowmetry (LDF) shows fluctuations in a blood flow in about 1 mm^3 of tissue based on a single-point technique measurement [25]. This method is mostly used for recording of perfusion in fingers during the attack of RP and the change of the blood perfusion after pharmacological interventions. Device head remains, however, attached to the point on the skin and any cutaneous irregularities may impair the read of underlying perfusion. Additionally, movements of fingers may produce artifacts in the record of the blood flow [26]. Combining of several single measurements over the surface of finger enables to measure perfusion across the finger. Laser Doppler perfusion imaging (LDPI) uses a moveable mirror that directs the laser beam on the different measurement allowing for raster scanning or line scanning of a surface. Obtained images are

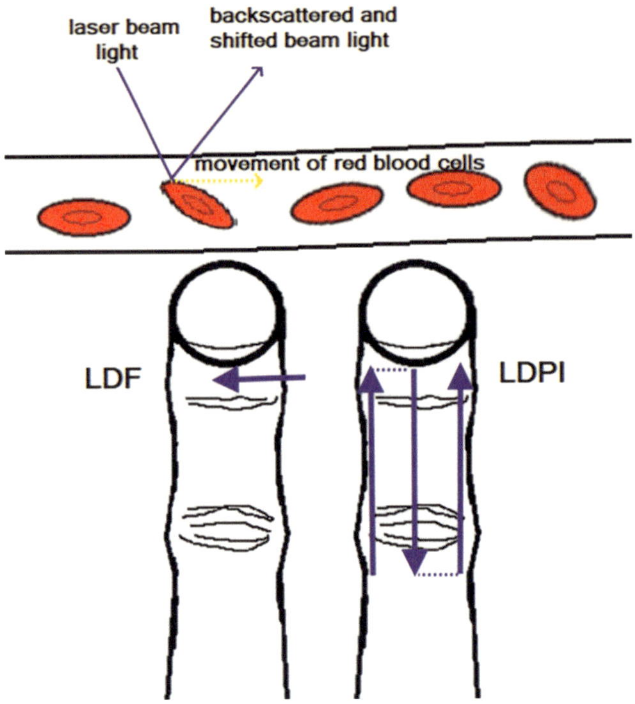

Figure 12.
Laser Doppler methods with a detection of backscattered laser beam light, which is shifted due to the movement of red blood cells. This can be laser Doppler flowmetry (LDF) with single point measurement or laser Doppler perfusion imaging (LDPI) with line or raster scanning.

composed of multiple pixels and displayed on the screen [25]. This imaging modality helps to analyze change in the perfusion of entire finger when evaluation of the risk for the development of digital tip ulcers is needed. Technique that does not require time-consuming scanning is laser speckle contrast analysis (LASCA), because it shows continuously perfusion in the hand. Laser Doppler methods and LASCA may seem different imaging techniques which developed separately, but a mathematical analysis shows that the two approaches are, in fact, identical. Illumination of a tissue leads herein to irregular backscattering of the laser light, which creates dark and light interference pattern (speckle pattern) [27]. CCD camera with a fixed exposure time records these changes in the speckle pattern as a motion. The speckle pattern is stationary when illuminated object remains static but moving red blood cells in a tissue produces blurring over time. The image is more blurred when there are more moving erythrocytes and the contrast between speckles decreases. Lack of movements means to a loss of blurring and therefore the contrast between speckles is large [25].

7. Infrared thermography

Imaging method that enables for indirect evaluation of the microvasculopathy is thermography. Skin surface emits infrared radiation (IR), which energy can be collected by lenses and converted to an electric signal, amplified and shown on a screen of thermal imaging camera. A colorful map of temperature distribution is created over the body surface and one may determine maximal, minimal and average temperature in a region of interest. These measurements can be done using both industrial and mobile thermal imaging cameras attached to smartphone [28].

A change in a local blood perfusion influences on IR and temperature, but it also depends on a body area and underlying inflammation [28–30]. One should remember to ensure right environmental conditions (e.g., room temperature 19–21 C, fixed humidity) and adaptation of patients not to disturb the measurements of IR. When there is the measurement of temperature distribution in hands, the patient should be asked to avoid smoking, coffee and alcohol drinking, hand washing, and moisturizing before testing not to force a change in IR emission [30, 31]. The recording should be performed perpendicularly to the dorsal aspect of hands (from the distance of 0.4–0.6 m), which are isolated from the background, for example, by the cork plate or gauze (**Figure 13**). To investigate nailfolds of finger II-V both hands should be positioned flat. The measure of temperature in nailfolds of thumbs seems to be preferentially performed in the fist, when thumbs lay on a cork plate or gauze and fingers II–V remain covered below (**Figure 14**). Regions of interests can be determined over the nailfolds, but measurements may include a gradient of temperatures between the center of the metacarpus and the nailfolds of separate fingers [32, 33].

Although there was found only moderate correlation between temperature measurements in nailfolds and the density of capillaries, thermography showed dependence of IR emission on capillaroscopic patterns in patients with SSc. One should remember that thermography measures IR emission from the portion of the tissue (3D space), whereas capillaroscopy quantifies density of vascular loops on a short distance (2D space) [32]. Thermography recently demonstrated differences in the control of temperature in hands between SSc patients with limited and diffuse cutaneous involvement [33]. Finally, thermography seems to be promising for the identification of fingers at then greater risk for the development of digital tip ulcers [32].

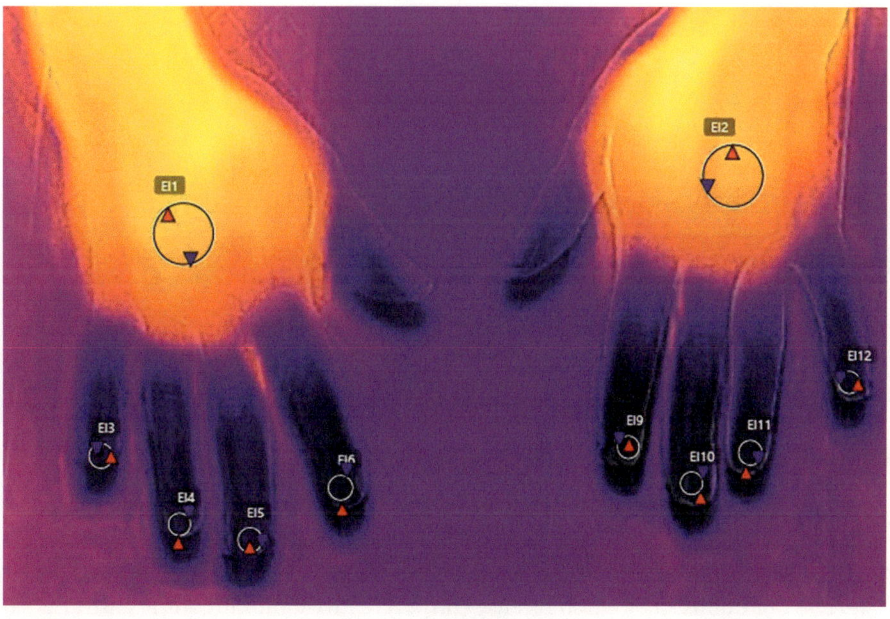

Figure 13.
Thermography of finger II–V performed with the use of FLIR T420 camera.

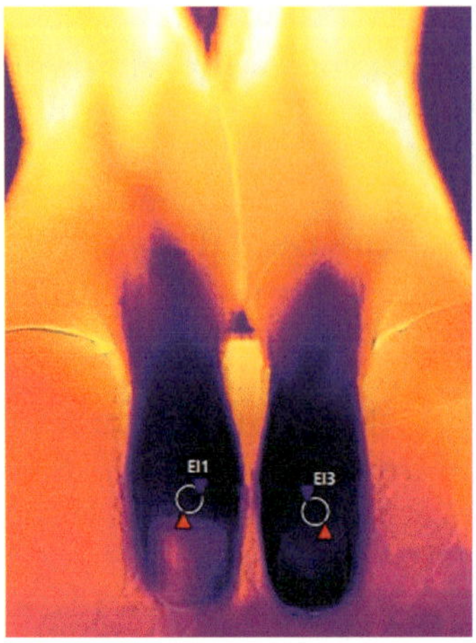

Figure 14.
Thermography of thumbs performed with the use of FLIR T420 camera.

Author details

Bartosz Miziołek*, Michał Szczepanek and Beata Bergler-Czop
Department of Dermatology, Medical University of Silesia, School of Medicine in Katowice, Poland

*Address all correspondence to: bmiziolek@gmail.com

References

[1] Smith V, Herrick AL, Ingegnoli F, Damjanov N, De Angelis R, Denton CP, et al. Standardisation of nailfold capillaroscopy for the assessment of patients with Raynaud's phenomenon and systemic sclerosis. Autoimmunity Reviews. 2020;**19**(3):102458

[2] Lombard WP. The blood pressur in the arterioles, capillaries, and small veins of the human skin. The American Journal of Physiology. 1912;**29**(3):335-362

[3] Brown GE, O'Leary PA. Skin capillaries in scleroderma. Archives of Internal Medicine (Chicago, Ill). 1925;**36**(1):73-88

[4] Maricq HR, LeRoy EC. Capillary blood flow in scleroderma. Bibliotheca Anatomica. 1973;**11**:352-358

[5] Maricq HR, LeRoy EC. Patterns of finger capillary abnormalities in connective tissue disease by "wide-field" microscopy. Arthritis and Rheumatism. 1973;**16**(5):619-628

[6] Maricq HR, Downey JA, LeRoy EC. Standstill of nailfold capillary blood flow during cooling in scleroderma and Raynaud's syndrome. Blood Vessels. 1976;**13**(6):338-349

[7] Minier T, Guiducci S, Bellando-Randone S, Bruni C, Lepri G, Czirják L, et al. Preliminary analysis of the very early diagnosis of systemic sclerosis (VEDOSS) EUSTAR multicentre study: Evidence for puffy fingers as a pivotal sign for suspicion of systemic sclerosis. Annals of the Rheumatic Diseases. 2014;**73**(12):2087-2093

[8] van den Hoogen F, Khanna D, Fransen J, Johnson SR, Baron M, Tyndall A, et al. 2013 classification criteria for systemic sclerosis: An American college of rheumatology/ European league against rheumatism collaborative initiative. Annals of the Rheumatic Diseases. 2013;**72**(11):1747-1755

[9] Aringer M, Costenbader K, Daikh D, Brinks R, Mosca M, Ramsey-Goldman R, et al. 2019 European League Against Rheumatism/American College of Rheumatology classification criteria for systemic lupus erythematosus. Annals of the Rheumatic Diseases. 2019;**78**(9):1151-1159

[10] Lundberg IE, Tjärnlund A, Bottai M, Werth VP, Pilkington C, de Visser M, et al. EULAR/ACR classification criteria for adult and juvenile idiopathic inflammatory myopathies and their major subgroups. Annals of the Rheumatic Diseases. 2017;**76**(12):1955-1964

[11] Smith V, Riccieri V, Pizzorni C, et al. Nailfold capillaroscopy for prediction of novel future severe organ involvement in systemic sclerosis. The Journal of Rheumatology. 2013;**40**:2023-2028

[12] Cutolo M, Sulli A, Pizzorni C, Accardo S. Nailfold videocapillaroscopy assessment of microvascular damage in systemic sclerosis. The Journal of Rheumatology. 2000;**27**:155-160

[13] Li N, Zang H, Sun H, Jiao X, Wang K, Liu TCT, et al. A Noninvasive accurate measurement of blood glucose levels with raman spectroscopy of blood in microvessels. Molecules. 2019;**24**(8):1500

[14] Fedorovich AA, Drapkina OM, Pronko KN, Sinopalnikov VI, Zemskov VM. Telemonitoring of capillary blood flow in the human skin:

New opportunities and prospects. Clinics and Practice. 2018;**15**(2):561-567

[15] Hurabielle C, Avouac J, Lepri G, de Risi T, Kahan A, Allanore Y. Skin telangiectasia and the identification of a subset of systemic sclerosis patients with severe vascular disease. Arthritis Care & Research (Hoboken). 2016;**68**(7):1021-1027

[16] Sekiyama JY, Camargo CZ, Eduardo LC, Kayser AC. Reliability of widefield nailfold capillaroscopy and videocapillaroscopy in the assessment of patients with raynaud's phenomenon. Arthritis Care & Research (Hoboken). 2013;**65**(11):1853-1861

[17] Grassi W, Rossella De Angelis R. Capillaroscopy: Questions and answers. Clinical Rheumatology. 2007;**26**(12):2009

[18] Miziołek B, Pieczyrak R, Polak K, Frątczak A, Jedlecka A, Grosicka A, et al. Role of short courses on nailfold capillaroscopy in obtaining abilities for the identification of microvasculopathy in patients with Raynaud's phenomenon. Skin Research and Technology. 2023;**29**(1):e13223

[19] Sha M, Griffin M, Denton CP, Butler PE. Sidestream Dark Field (SDF) imaging of oral microcirculation in the assessment of systemic sclerosis. Microvascular Research. 2019;**126**:103890

[20] Miranda S, Armengol G, Le Besnerais M, Lévesque H, Benhamou Y. New insights into systemic sclerosis related microcirculatory dysfunction by assessment of sublingual microcirculation and vascular glycocalyx layer. Results from a preliminary study. Microvascular Research. 2015;**99**:72-77

[21] Ranjbar M, Rothe M, Klapa S, Lange T, Prasuhn M, Grisanti S, et al. Evaluation of choroidal substructure perfusion in patients affected by systemic sclerosis: An optical coherence tomography angiography study. Scandinavian Journal of Rheumatology. 2020;**49**(2):141-145

[22] Rommel F, Prangel D, Prasuhn M, Grisanti S, Ranjbar M. Correlation of retinal and choroidal microvascular impairment in systemic sclerosis. Orphanet Journal of Rare Diseases. 2021;**16**(1):27

[23] Abignano G, Aydin SZ, Castillo-Gallego C, Liakouli V, Woods D, Meekings A, et al. Virtual skin biopsy by optical coherence tomography: The first quantitative imaging biomarker for scleroderma. Annals of the Rheumatic Diseases. 2013;**72**(11):1845-1851

[24] Abignano G, Green L, Eng S, Emery P, Del Galdo F. Nailfold microvascular imaging by dynamic optical coherence tomography in systemic sclerosis: A case-controlled pilot study. The Journal of Investigative Dermatology. 2022;**142**(4):1050-1057

[25] Eriksson S, Nilsson J, Sturesson C. Non-invasive imaging of microcirculation: A technology review. Medical Devices (Auckland). 2014;7:445-452

[26] Herrick AL, Dinsdale G, Murray A. New perspectives in the imaging of Raynaud's phenomenon. European Journal of Rheumatology. 2020;7(Suppl 3):S212-S221

[27] Briers JD. Laser doppler, speckle and related techniques for blood perfusion mapping and imaging. Physiological Measurement. 2001;**22**:R35-R66

[28] Lahiri BB, Bagavathiappan S, Jayakumar T, Philip J. Medical applications of infrared thermography: A review.

Infrared Physics & Technology. 2012;**55**(4):221-235

[29] Ludwig N, Formenti D, Gargano M, Alberti G. Skin temperature evaluation by infrared thermography: Comparison of image analysis methods. Infrared Physics & Technology. 2014;**62**:1-6

[30] Lis-Święty A, Miziołek B, Ranosz-JanickaI,Bierzyńska-MacyszynG, Brzezińska-Wcisło L. Thermal imaging and dermoscopy for detecting inflammation in frontal fibrosing alopecia. Journal of Cosmetic Dermatology. 2018;**17**(2):268-273

[31] Szczepanek M, Frątczak A, Polak K, Lis-Święty A. Narrow-band reflectance spectrophotometry and infrared thermography for assessment of skin lesions in localized scleroderma. Journal of the European Academy of Dermatology and Venereology. 2022;**36**(12):2451-2458

[32] Miziołek B, Lis-Święty A, Skrzypek-Salamon A, Brzezińska-Wcisło L. Correlation between the infrared thermogram and microvascular abnormalities of the nailfold in patients with systemic sclerosis. Postepy Dermatologii I Alergologii. 2021;**38**(2):115-122

[33] Miziołek B, Lis-Święty A, Kucharz E, Pieczyrak R, Polak K, Szczepanek M, et al. Clinical assessment of patients with systemic sclerosis: Is there a place for thermography? Archives of Dermatological Research. 2023;**315**(3):387-393

Chapter 5

Assessment of Lung Involvement and Prognostic Value of the 6-Minute Walking Test for Pulmonary Involvement in Patients with Systemic Sclerosis

Mariela Geneva-Popova, Stanislava Popova-Belova, Sanie Dzambasova, Velichka Popova and Vladimir Hodhzev

Abstract

Systemic sclerosis (SSc) is a chronic multisystemic immune-mediated disease with multifactorial etiology, variable clinical symptomatology, and treatment with limited efficacy. In recent years, biomarkers of SSc and predictors of disease progression and organ's involvement have been intensively studied in order to identify the most appropriate therapeutic choice for the patients. The lungs are frequently affected in the pathological processes in patients with SSc, and this is often the main cause of death in these patients due to involvement of the lung parenchyma or pulmonary vessels. In daily clinical practice, it is necessary to have a relatively accurate and easily reproducible methods for assessing functional capacity of this organ. The comparative characterization of the "field tests" shows that the 6-minute walk test is a convenient test for assessing functional activity in patients with moderately severe and severe connective tissue diseases. It is easy to administer, well reproducible, acceptable to patients, sensitive to therapeutic procedures. The 6MWT is the method of choice for assessing functional capacity in systemic connective tissue diseases such as SSc with pulmonary involvement, and the pilot study shows that it can be used as a novel biomarker for assessing of pulmonary involvement.

Keywords: 6-minute walk test, systemic sclerosis, interstitial lung disease, pulmonary hypertension, biomarkers

1. Introduction

Systemic sclerosis (SSc) is a chronic multisystemic immune-mediated disease with a multifactorial etiology, variable clinical symptomatology, and treatment with limited efficacy [1–3]. SSc is a disease of significant social importance, as patients suffering from this disease have health, economic, social and family problems [4–6].

SSc remains one of the challenging disease in rheumatology. Despite decades of intensive clinical and basic research, as well as dozens of clinical trials, the causes and pathophysiological mechanisms of the disease remain largely unrecognized. In real clinical medicine, there is still a lack of fully effective therapies to cure all affected tissues and organs from the pathological process [7, 8].

Chifflot et al. studied the incidence and prevalence of SSc in adults [9]. According to their publication, based on a systematic review of the literature, the authors found that the prevalence of SSc ranges from 7/million to 489/million and its incidence from 0.6/million/year to 122/million/year [9]. According to the authors, there is a trend towards an increase in the incidence of SSc over time. The authors conclude that there is a need to continue research into various aspects of the disease [9]. The incidence and prevalence of SSc vary widely depending on geographic location and analysis methods.

There has been an increasing trend in the incidence of SSc over time [3]. Overall survival has improved over the past few decades and is approximately 12 years from diagnosis [3, 9]. Nevertheless, a major problem is still high mortality due to multiorgan involvement, and lung disease has emerged as the leading cause of death [5].

In recent years, biomarkers of SSc and the possibilities of distinguishing its subtypes, predictors of disease progression and intra-organ involvement have been intensively studied in order to identify the most appropriate therapeutic choice for the specific patient [10].

The pathogenesis of SSc is complex, multifactorial and not fully understood. Evidence of three processes can be found in any patient with SSc - vascular injury, immune dysfunction and tissue remodeling. These processes do not occur in isolation, but are interconnected and mutually modulated [11, 12]. The triad of vasculopathy, autoimmunity/inflammation, and connective tissue remodeling underlies the clinical and laboratory manifestations of scleroderma, ranging from clinical manifestation of Raynaud's phenomenon, autoantibody synthesis, or pulmonary fibrosis [13]. Vascular and endothelial damage are early and possibly primary events in the evolution of the disease and can be detected on initial examination in most patients. While initially vascular damage is associated with reversible functional changes, progressive and irreversible structural vascular changes increase over time. This is followed by progressive vascular damage with obliteration of small and medium-sized arteries in multiple vascular beds and associated activation of thrombotic and coagulation cascades. Reduced blood supply leads to tissue hypoxia, ischemia and its complications [14, 15].

According to Guiducci et al., damage to the vascular wall is characterized by the formation of megacapillaries and avascular zones [15]. The authors reported that decreased capillary density leads to clinical manifestations such as digital ulcers [15]. Guiducci et al., reported that despite reduced blood flow and reduced levels of oxygen partial pressure, there is paradoxically no evidence of sufficient angiogenesis in the skin of patients with SSc [15]. Angiogenesis is severely impaired in SSc, as evidenced by nail videocapillaroscopy changes, vessel damage develops progressively from early to late stages [15]. Many of the severe internal organ complications of SSc are vascular, including pulmonary arterial hypertension (PAH) and scleroderma renal crisis. Structural vascular damage occurs in many vascular beds and contributes to pulmonary, renal, cardiac, and gastrointestinal complications. Vascular damage has a role in the activation of the innate and acquired immune systems and contributes directly or indirectly to tissue fibrosis [16, 17].

Immune dysfunction induces synthesis of highly specific autoantibodies and activation of fibroblasts in most parenchymal tissues and around blood vessels [18].

Immune dysfunction in SSc is characterized by the activation and recruitment of immune cells (T cells, B cells, dendritic cells, mast cells, macrophages and others) and the production of autoantibodies (anti-TOPO-I, kinetochore proteins, RNA polymerase enzyme (anti-RNAP III), ribonuclear proteins (anti-U11/U12 RNP, anti-U1 RNP, anti-U3 RNP, nucleolar antigens (anti-Th/To, anti-NOR 90, anti-Ku, antiRuvBL1/2, and anti-PM/Scl and others) and cytokines (transforming growth factor (TGF)-β, interleukin (IL)-6 and IL-4, chemokines). Immune dysfunction in SSc leads to significant matrix synthesis and deposition that disrupts the architecture and function of the affected organ (lung, spleen, liver, skin, heart, peri-articular soft tissues) [19].

The lungs are frequently affected in SSc patients and are the main cause of mortality in patients with the disease [20, 21]. Current studies have investigated gene expression in the lungs of patients with SSc, analyzing patterns associated with PAH and interstitial lung disease (ILD) [21, 22].

According to Distler et al., ILD is the leading cause of death in SSc [21]. In their article, the authors report that there are no valid biomarkers for predicting the onset of SSc-ILD, although anti-topoisomerase I autoantibodies and several inflammatory markers are candidate biomarkers that need further evaluation [21]. Again in the same article, they reveal that auscultation of the chest, the presence of dyspnea, and pulmonary function testing are important diagnostic tools, but they lack sensitivity for detecting early IBD [21]. Therefore, baseline screening with high-resolution computed tomography (HRCT) is required to confirm the diagnosis of SSc-ILD [21]. It is important to monitor patients with SSc-ILD for signs of disease progression, although there is no consensus on which diagnostic tools to use or how often monitoring should be performed.

According to Distler et al., there is no valid definition of disease progression of SSc-ILD. The authors suggest that a decrease in forced vital capacity (FVC) from baseline of ≥10%, or a decline in FVC of 5–9% in association with a decrease in the diffusing capacity of the lung for carbon monoxide of ≥15% should be counted as progression of the disease [21]. According to the same authors, patients with SSc should be analyzed every 12–24 months to monitor disease progression/regression.

SSc-related PAH shows increased expression of inflammatory genes [21, 22]. A significant number of genes with increased expression are shared between SSc-related pulmonary fibrosis (SSc-PF) and idiopathic pulmonary fibrosis (IPF), as well as SSc-PAH and idiopathic PAH, highlighting possible overlaps in pathogenetic mechanisms between these two, which sometimes occur together in SSc [23–25].

Increased knowledge about systemic sclerosis and improved diagnostic methods in recent decades have led to the possibility of diagnosing systemic sclerosis in earlier stages of the disease and its earlier treatment. This matters for each patient and increases the quality of care for them by the rheumatologist [26–29].

2. Serum biomarkers for pulmonary fibrosis

Markers of organ-specific fibrosis would be of great clinical importance because pulmonary involvement is a severe complication of SSc [26]. Intensive research efforts have focused on identifying biomarkers of lung involvement early in the course of the disease and also as prognostic factors for response to treatment [26]. Transforming growth factor is a pleiotropic factor that regulates various biological processes such as cell development, tissue regeneration, immune responses, and others. TGF is required for lung homeostasis [30], and is important for epithelial-mesenchymal interactions during lung morphogenesis and alveolarization. Upregulation of TGF-β ligands is observed in pulmonary fibrosis, emphysema, bronchial asthma, etc. TGF-β regulates multiple cellular processes, such as suppression of epithelial cell growth, alveolar epithelial cell differentiation, fibroblast activation, and extracellular matrix organization matrix. These effects are closely related to tissue remodeling in pulmonary fibrosis [30]. TGF-β1 has a central role in the pathogenesis of fibrotic diseases and is a candidate biomarker in SSc [31, 32]. Higher levels of TGF-β1 have been found in the serum of patients with SSc compared with healthy controls [31].

Other candidate biomarkers for lung involvement have been identified and are the Krebs von den Lungen-6 antigen (KL-6) and protein surfactants A and D (PS-A and D) [33]. Serum levels of KL-6 and PS-D are significantly higher in SSc patients compared to healthy subjects and are associated with ILD activity as measured by lung function and high-resolution computed tomography - HRCT [34]. Serum levels of KL-6 are closely related to changes in FVC, making it a promising marker for the follow-up of ILD activity after treatment, and high serum levels of PS-D are a predictor of FVC decline in dynamics [34] and are in close association with pulmonary fibrosis [33, 34]. The two biomarkers KL-6 and PS-D correlate and show similar sensitivity and specificity for the diagnosis of ILD [35, 36]. In the Scleroderma Lung Study group, baseline PS-D and KL-6 levels were examined in patients with and without alveolitis as determined by HRCT. Higher serum levels of both biomarkers have been confirmed in SSc patients compared to healthy controls, as well as in SSc patients with alveolitis compared to those without alveolitis [36].

A biomarker for lung involvement is interleukin-6 (IL-6), which is a pleiotropic cytokine associated with Th2 lymphocytes [37, 38]. Despite the key importance of IL-6 in physiological processes, elevated levels have been described in several lung diseases [38] as well as in the serum of patients with SSc, and there is a significant correlation between them and the results of instrumental studies of the lung and cardiovascular system [38].

In the exploratory analysis, only serum IL-6 among IL-8, IL-10, CCL2, CXCL10, vascular endothelial growth factors (VEGFs), fibroblast growth factor-2 and CX3CL1 was shown to be an independent predictor of respiratory failure decline in patients with systemic sclerosis. At a value of 7.7 pg./mL, serum IL-6 predicted decline in FVC (HR 2.58) and DLCO (HR 3.2) in the first year and predicted death in the first 30 months (HR 2.69). In SSc-ILD, serum levels of IL-6 appear to predict early disease progression [39]. Serum levels of another pleiotropic cytokine, IL-15, a T- and B-lymphocyte survival and growth factor, are associated with impaired lung function in SSc [40]. Th17 lymphocyte-associated IL-17A and IL-23 levels are elevated in SSc and are associated with the presence of ILD [41]. Circulating IL-22- and IL-17-producing T cells are increased in patients with SSc-ILD compared with those without ILD [40].

Truchetet et al. found increased frequency of circulating Th22 in addition to Th17 and Th2 lymphocytes in systemic sclerosis and this is with association with interstitial lung disease [41, 42].

3. Pulmonary function tests

Pulmonary function tests are not a sensitive screening method for determining lung involvement in SSc, therefore, using only this test at follow-up may miss a number of patients with ILD [43]. In the context of ILD, involvement of more than one-third of the lung parenchyma and the presence of reduced FVC early in the disease classifies patients at higher risk of disease progression, thus identifying a subset of patients with greater potential benefits of immunosuppression [44]. In patients with milder disease, it is more difficult to establish a cut off for the risk of progression. After multivariate logistic regression analysis of two cohorts, lower peripheral oxygen saturation (SpO2) < 94% after the 6-minute walking test (6MWT) and the presence of arthritis at any time during the follow-up period were found to be independent predictors of progression of ILD at 1 year. Based on this, a prediction model was developed that was able to stratify the risk of mild ILD progression with a positive predictive value of 91.7% and a specificity of 98.6% [45].

4. Lung ultrasound (LUS)

In recent years, much data has become available on the role of transthoracic lung ultrasound (TTUS) in the evaluation of various lung conditions [46]. Although the role of ultrasoundgraphy (US) has been described in detail in the literature, in recent years the validity of the technique in the assessment of pulmonary fibrosis in patients with SSc has been investigated [46]. Lung ultrasonography has established itself as a noninvasive, inexpensive, easily applicable, radiation-free method with high sensitivity and specificity for diagnosis, even in the early preclinical phase of pulmonary fibrosis [46, 47]. This methodology has been established as a technique for evaluating superficial chest structures such as pleural effusion, pleural and subpleural findings (tumors), or pleural motion for the diagnosis of pneumothorax, as well as for ultrasound-guided manipulations [46, 47]. In one of the first publications on the application of ultrasonography in patients with diffuse parenchymal lung disease, a close relationship was demonstrated between the diagnosis of ILD and the three special sonographic findings: number of B-lines, pleural changes (roughness, thickening, fragmentation) and subpleural changes [48].

The ultrasound characteristic of pulmonary fibrosis consists in the detection and quantification of the so-called US comets (B-lines). B-lines are defined as discrete laser-like vertical hyperechoic reverberations emanating from the pleural line, from US beam reflection from the thickened subpleural interlobular septa (described as "comet tails"), reaching the bottom of the screen without fading, and move synchronously with lung movement [48].

Ultrasound B-lines are an excellent noninvasive method for assessing ILD in patients with SSc [49]. In a single-center study of 40 patients with SSc, the excellent correlation between the number of B-lines assessed by US and the Warrick score was confirmed (Spearman rho: 0.958, p = 0.0001). ROC curve analysis revealed that 10 US B-lines was the cut-off with the highest risk of the probability of significant SSc-ILD [49]. Thus, the detection of at least 10 B-lines is highly predictive of the presence of SSc-ILD on HRCT. In patients with SSc, evaluation of the lungs as the first-line imaging tool can be an effective means of determining the most appropriate time to perform HRCT of the chest [49].

The lung in patients with rheumatic diseases [50]. The author studied 30 patients with SSc and found that the number of B-lines was higher in Scl-70 positive than in negative patients [50]. In the following years, other researchers proved the correlation between B-lines and HRCT result [51]. The specificity and sensitivity of ultrasonography with respect to HRCT were found to be 70% and 85% for cardiac probe and 60% and 85% for linear [51].

In healthy individuals, the pleural line is visualized as a hyperechoic line resulting from the reflection of the parietal and visceral pleura. The normal pleural line is thin, continuous, and without nodular thickening. Pleural line thickening >2.8 mm was considered pathologic [52].

The degree of distribution of pleural irregularities and B-lines compared with clinical, spirometric and DLCO indices, systems assessments (Warrick and Wells) and quantification of ILD severity using HRCT demonstrates that pleural assessment is an equally reliable finding in the diagnosis and stratification of severity according to the degree of ILD [53].

5. High-resolution computed tomography (HRCT) of the lung

Conventional chest radiography is widely used as the first-choice tool for the imaging assessment of pulmonary fibrosis, but low sensitivity in the early stages limits its use in daily clinical practice [54–56]. HRCT is a highly sensitive diagnostic method for the routine detection and evaluation of pulmonary complications of patients with SSc and is the gold standard method for the diagnosis of both SSc-related ILD [46] and for the evaluation of pulmonary involvement—early changes and subclinical involvement, but the routine its application is limited by high cost and exposure to high doses of ionizing radiation [56].

All these methods significantly indicate the state of the patient's pulmonary involvement and correlate very well with each other, but require expensive equipment and a trained specialist in the relevant field.

6. 6-minute walking test (6MWT)

In daily clinical practice, it is necessary to have a relatively accurate and easily reproducible method for assessing the patient's functional capacity, which would reflect his condition to a significant extent.

"Physical capacity" (fitness, performance) represents the body's ability to successfully perform physical activity without applying excessive stress and within safe limits. Physical capacity is a complex indicator of the general functional state of a person and his motor abilities. It depends on physical development, gender, age and hereditary predispositions [57, 58].

There are different methods for objectifying functional physical capacity. Some are high-tech and provide a comprehensive assessment of all systems relevant to physical activity, while others provide only basic information but require simpler technology and are easier to implement. The choice of functional testing method should be based on clinical requirements and available options [58, 59].

Methods for measuring physical capacity can generally be divided into two groups - laboratory and field. Laboratory conditions allow maximal, symptom-limited tests to be performed using a cycle ergometer or treadmill with parallel measurement of ventilation parameters, hemodynamics and important metabolic parameters. They provide useful information about limiting factors and the maximum load that an individual can reach and allow precise analysis of the load/response relationship, but are difficult to perform in disabled patients [60]. These tests are known in the literature as cardiopulmonary exercise tests [60].

Exercise walking, on the other hand, is an inexpensive and accessible means of determining exercise tolerance in the absence of resources to perform cardiopulmonary exercise testing [61].

Walking tests are also called "field tests" because they are conducted outside a laboratory. Field tests include the step test and walking tests. Despite its simplicity and accessibility, the step test has failed to establish itself permanently in clinical practice, due to a lack of consensus regarding its standardization in human patients [61]. In turn, walking tests are divided into time-limited (time walk tests) and shuttle walk tests (shuttle walk tests).

For the first time in the early 1960s, a simplified test for assessing functional capacity was proposed by Balke [61]. The twelve-minute test was first applied by Cooper K. in 1968 [62]. He found that the distance covered in 12 minutes by young men correlated excellently ($r = 0.9$) with maximal oxygen consumption (VO2max.) measured by treadmill exercise [62].

In pulmonology, a simplified test to assess functional lung capacity was first introduced by McGavin et al. in 1976, who modified this outdoor running test into a 12-min indoor walking format to measure exercise tolerance in chronic bronchitis patients [63]. An interval of 12 "working" minutes is associated with significantly increased demands in sick individuals and in 1982 Butland et al. divides the walking test into 2- and 6-minute modules [62]. While the 6MWT correlates well with the 12-min test, the short-term 2-MWT may overestimate physical capacity in well-motivated subjects [62]. It is argued that the 6MWT is easy to perform, well tolerated, and adequately reflects daily activities for functional diagnostic needs [62].

The 6MWT is a practically simple test that requires the presence of a corridor 30 meters long, without special equipment and technical training. Walking is an activity performed daily by all but the most severely ill patients. This test measures the distance a patient can walk quickly on a smooth, hard surface in 6 minutes. The test evaluates the global and integrated response of all systems involved in motor activity – respiratory and cardiovascular, systemic circulation, blood, neuromuscular units and muscle metabolism. The test does not provide information about the function of the various organs and systems involved in the motor act and about the mechanism of motor limitation, as does the cardiopulmonary physical test. The 6MWT assesses the submaximal level of functional capacity [64].

Most patients do not reach maximal physical capacity during the 6MWT – they have control over walking intensity and can rest during the test. Because most daily activities are performed at submaximal exertion, the 6MWT better reflects daily functional exertion.

6MWT, it is reliable in the majority of patients with SSc. The 6MWT is a good basis for comparing values in the individual patient at different time points, rather than relying on reference standards, because the general population cannot provide a reliable comparison in these individuals [65, 66]. Performing the 6MWT on SSc patients twice, at a minimum interval of 3 months, showed strong reproducibility of this test and indicated that mRSS, arthralgias and tendon friction, FVC, DLCO, left ventricular EF were associated with lower 6MWT [65, 66]. Given that 6MWT at first examination is an independent predictor of overall mortality and SSc-related mortality, this test is considered useful for assessing overall prognosis in patients with SSc [67]. To detect progression of pulmonary fibrosis, reduced HRCT can be an alternative to standard HRCT and be used in patients with SSc to detect early progression of pulmonary fibrosis [68].

The indications for conducting 6MWT are many, as it is often used for pre- and post-operative comparison of results in lung transplants, lung resection, lung parenchyma reduction, COPD, lung rehabilitation, heart failure, and others. It is very often used in determining the functional status of patients with COPD, HF, peripheral vascular disease, cystic fibrosis, in adult patients. Based on the results of the 6MWT test, it is also possible to make a prediction about the survival and mortality of these diseases [66].

There are also absolute contraindications for conducting the 6MWT are unstable angina and myocardial infarction in the previous month. Relative contraindications are resting heart rate > 120 bpm, systolic blood pressure > 180 mmHg, and diastolic blood pressure > 100 mmHg [66].

Stable angina on exercise is not an absolute contraindication for the 6MWT, but in patients with these symptoms the test should be performed after antianginal medication and in the presence of nitrates during the test. Each patient determines their own exercise intensity, and the test (without electrocardiographic monitoring) has been performed in very elderly patients [64] and patients with heart failure and cardiomyopathy without serious adverse effects [63].

The contraindications listed were used by the study investigators based on their perceptions of the safety of the 6MWT, but the occurrence of adverse side effects when performing the 6MWT in these patients is unknown; therefore, it is about relative contraindications.

Preparing for the test:

1. The test must be carried out in a place where it is possible to apply appropriate and timely emergency medical care.

2. The test should be conducted with the availability of emergency medication.

3. The test taker must be qualified to perform cardiopulmonary resuscitation, with proficiency in advanced CPR techniques desirable.

4. It is not necessary to have a doctor present during the test. The doctor appoints the test to be performed; the presence of a doctor is at individual discretion.

5. If the patient is on chronic oxygen therapy, oxygen should be administered at a standard dose or per protocol. Reasons for immediate termination of the 6MWT may include: chest pain, intolerable dyspnea, limb cramps, vertigo, profuse sweating, or pallor [66, 67].

If the test is stopped for any of these reasons, the patient should sit or lie down depending on the severity of the condition and the risk of syncope. Blood pressure, pulse rate, oxygen saturation should be measured and a medical examination should be performed. Administration of oxygen is appropriate [66, 67].

7. Technical aspects of 6MWT

The 6MWT should be performed indoors – a long, straight, level, enclosed corridor with a hard surface. If the weather is suitable, the test can also be performed outside. The length of the corridor should be 30 meters. The corridor must be marked along its length every 3 meters. The end point must be marked (eg with an orange sign). The starting line, which marks the beginning and end of each 60-meter transition, must be marked with a bright tape. The shorter corridor requires patients to change direction multiple times, reducing the 6MWD value. Most studies used a 30-m corridor, but some used a 20- or 50-m corridor [69]. A multicenter study found no significant effect of corridor length (9 to 50 meters) [69].

DOI: http://dx.doi.org/10.5772/intechopen.1002989

Necessary equipment includes – timer, mechanical counter, two small cones to mark the end of the corridor, chair that can be easily moved while walking, patient data form, oxygen source, sphygmomanometer, telephone, defibrillator.

Measurements:

1. Repeat testing should be performed at the same time of day to minimize time-of-day variability.

2. No "warming up" should be done before the test.

3. The patient must stand or sit in a chair placed near the starting position at least 10 minutes before the start of the test. During this time, contraindications should be checked, pulse and blood pressure should be measured, and shoes and clothing should be checked for comfort. The first page of the form is filled out.

4. Pulse oximetry is optional. When performed, baseline heart rate and oxygen saturation (SpO2) were recorded, following the manufacturer's instructions to amplify the signal and minimize motor artifacts. The pulse should be regular and the quality of the oximetry signal good [69].

5. In the standing position of the patient, dyspnea and general fatigue are measured according to the Borg scale (0 Absence, 0.5 – very, very weak (almost imperceptible), 1 very weak, 2 – weak, 3 – moderate, 4 – moderately severe, 5 – heavy, 6, 7 - very heavy, 8, 9, 10 – very, very heavy (maximum)

At the beginning of the 6-minute test, the scale is shown to the patient with the words: "Please rate your degree of shortness of breath on the scale" and then: "Please rate your degree of fatigue on this scale." At the end of the study, the patient is reminded of the values he chose and asked to rate his dyspnea and fatigue again.

1. The counter is reset and the timer is set to 6 minutes. The patient stands at the starting line.

2. The patient is given instructions aimed at standardizing the examination and avoiding errors. In addition, it is necessary that the patient be trained and given detailed information about possible difficulties that he would have when performing it.

3. The patient is positioned at the starting line. The technician remains near the starting line during the test and does not accompany the patient. The timer starts as soon as the patient starts walking.

4. The technician must not speak during the test. The same tone of voice is used to pronounce standard phrases.

5. After the test, the Borg's dyspnea and fatigue are recorded and the patient is asked: "Is there anything that would prevent you from walking a greater distance?"

6. When using a pulse oximeter, measure the SpO2 pulse rate, then remove the sensor.

7. The number of laps is recorded in the form.

8. The additional distance is marked (the meters traveled from the last incomplete lap are added) using the markers with which the corridor is mapped. The total distance traveled is calculated, rounded to the nearest meter and recorded on the form.

9. At the beginning and at the end of the 6-minute test, the scale is shown to the patient with the words: "Please rate your degree of shortness of breath on the scale" and then: "Please rate your degree of fatigue on this scale."

Only standardized phrases should be used during the test. Encouragement significantly increases the distance traveled. The reproducibility of tests with and without encouragement was similar. Encouragement every minute with standardized phrases is recommended [66, 69].

Among the factors lowering the value of 6MWD are short stature, advanced age, increased body weight, female gender, impaired cognitive function, shorter corridor (more turns), various pulmonary and cardiovascular diseases, musculoskeletal disease and others [69].

When the patient is tall, male, informed in advance about the nature of the test and highly motivated, we can respectively expect higher values for 6MWD [69].

8. Interpretation of functional status

There are still no standard reference values derived from healthy populations. These values can be calculated based on the results in healthy people of the same age. For them, a distance covered between 400 and 700 m is considered the norm, but there are various publications in which this value differs by about 30% among different researchers [70, 71].

Age, height, weight, and gender independently affect the 6MWT value in healthy subjects, and these factors should be taken into account when interpreting the results of single tests to determine functional status. A low 6MWD value is not specific and has no diagnostic value [70, 71].

The comparative characteristic of "field tests" shows that the 6MWT is a convenient test for assessing functional activity in patients with moderate and severe diseases. It is easy to administer, well reproducible, acceptable to patients, sensitive to therapeutic procedures and very well related to daily activities. Currently, the 6MWT is the test of choice when functional walking tests are to be applied for clinical and research purposes.

Garin and colleagues investigated the factors that influence 6MWT in patients with SSc - interstitial lung disease (ILD), SSc-pulmonary hypertension (PH) and idiopathic pulmonary fibrosis (IPF). They studied 48 patients with IPF, 33 patients with SSc-ILD, 13 with SSc-PH, 19 with both SSc-ILD and SSc-PH (SSc-Both), and 15 with SSc without ILD or PH (SSc-Neither either) and found that mean 6MWT did not differ between groups [72].

Someya and colleagues studied the cardiac hemodynamic response during exercise in 59 patients with systemic sclerosis and 27 age- and sex-matched healthy controls using a 6MWTt with a noninvasive impedance cardiograph [73]. The authors found that stroke volume and cardiac output in patients with systemic sclerosis were significantly lower than in controls at rest and at the end of the 6-minute walk test, and the distance traveled was significantly shorter in patients.

Someya and colleagues concluded that impaired stroke volume in patients with systemic sclerosis was observed at rest and during exercise, and factors related to the cardiac response appeared to be pulmonary function and the degree of pulmonary hypertension [73].

Vandecasteele et al. investigated interstitial lung disease (ILD) and pulmonary arterial hypertension (PAH) in patients with SSc, as they considered that although the 6MWT is used to assess ILD and PAH in clinical practice, no data are available for it and oxygen desaturation in SSc patients without ILD and PAH. The authors analyzed prospectively collected 6MWT data at baseline and 6-month follow-up of 300 consecutive patients with SSc [74].

Vandecasteele et al. found that the mean 6MWT of 165 SSc patients without ILD and PAH who performed the 6MWT at baseline or at the 6-month visit was 484 ± 93 m [74].

Vandecasteele et al. concluded that in SSc without ILD and PAH, 6MWD and oxygen desaturation were clinically stable over a 6-month period. The DcSSc subgroup walked less than the LSSc and LcSSc subgroups [74].

Sanges and colleagues investigated the 6MWT in the evaluation of patients with SSc and assessed various disease parameters [75]. Their data were systematically collected during a comprehensive standardized assessment that included a 6-minute walk test, clinical assessment, biological results, pulmonary function tests, transthoracic echocardiography, composite scores (European Scleroderma Study Group Activity Index, assessment of Medsger severity, Health Assessment Questionnaire-Disability Index (HAQ-DI)) and treatments [75].

Sanges et al. concluded that 6MWT was independently associated with baseline heart rate and its variability, suggesting that pulmonary vasculopathy may have a greater impact on functional limitation than parenchymal involvement; and with global markers of disease activity and patient disability. These results provide clinicians with additional insight into how to interpret 6MWD in the context of SSc [75].

The 6MWT is the method of choice for assessing functional capacity in systemic connective tissue diseases with pulmonary involvement [64, 70–74].

In routine practice, functional and imaging methods are used to confirm and assess the extent of lung involvement. In daily clinical practice, it is necessary to have a relatively accurate and easily reproducible method for assessing functional capacity, which would significantly reflect the patient's condition. The comparative characterization of the "field tests" shows that the 6-minute walk test is a convenient test for assessing functional activity in patients with moderately severe and severe connective tissue diseases. It is easy to administer, well reproducible, acceptable to patients, sensitive to therapeutic procedures and very well related to daily activities. Currently, the 6-minute walk test is the test of choice when functional walking tests are to be applied for clinical and research purposes.

The 6-minute walk test is the method of choice for assessing functional capacity in systemic connective tissue diseases with pulmonary involvement, and the pilot study shows that it can be used as a novel biomarker for assessing pulmonary involvement in patients with systemic connective tissue diseases [64, 71–74].

Future trends in the field of SSc, also outlined by EULAR, include validation of biomarkers for early diagnosis, subgroup classification, predictors of different organ involvement, identification of prognostic biomarkers as well as therapeutic efficacy biomarkers, some of which are likely to be and 6MWD.

According to our pilot study, 6MWT provides information regarding functional capacity, response to therapy and prognosis in patients with SSc and desaturation during a test an important prognostic indicator for patients.

Author details

Mariela Geneva-Popova[1*], Stanislava Popova-Belova[1], Sanie Dzambasova[1], Velichka Popova[2] and Vladimir Hodhzev[3]

1 Faculty of Medicine, Propedeutics of Internal Diseases, General Hospital "Sveti Georgi" Plovdiv, Rheumatology, Medical University, Plovdiv, Bulgaria

2 Faculty of Medicine, Propedeutics of Internal Diseases, General Hospital "Kaspela" Plovdiv, Rheumatology, Medical University, Plovdiv, Bulgaria

3 Department of Internal Diseases, Faculty of Medicine, General Hospital "Sveti Georgi" Plovdiv, Pulmonology, Medical University, Plovdiv, Bulgaria

*Address all correspondence to: genevapopova@yahoo.com

References

[1] Varga J, Trojanowska M, Kuwana M. Pathogenesis of systemic sclerosis: Recent insights of molecular and cellular mechanisms and therapeutic opportunities. Journal of Scleroderma Relates Disorders. 2017;**2**:137-152

[2] Mayes M. Scleroderma epidemiology. Rheumatic Diseases Clinics of North America. 2003;**29**(2):239-254. DOI: 10.1016/S0889-857X(03)00022-X

[3] Bernatsky S, Joseph L, Pineau C, Belisle P, Hudson M, Clarke A. Scleroderma prevalence: Demographic variations in a population-based sample. Arthritis and Rheumatism. 2009;**61**(3):400-404

[4] Bhattacharyya S, Wei J, Varga J. Understanding fibrosis in systemic sclerosis: Shifting paradigm, emerging opportunities. Nature Reviews Rheumatology. 2012;**8**(1):42-54

[5] Steen V, Medsger T. Changes in causes of death in systemic sclerosis, 1972-2002. Annals of the Rheumatic Diseases. 2007;**66**(7):940-944

[6] Kahaleh B, Mulligan-Kehoe M. Mechanisms of vascular disease. In: Varga J, Denton CP, Wigley FM, editors. Scleroderma: From Pathogenesis to Comprehensive Management. London: Springer-Verlag; 2012. pp. 227-246

[7] Volkmann E, Tashkin D. Treatment of systemic sclerosis-related interstitial lung disease: A review of existing and emerging therapies. Annals of the American Thoracic Society. 2016;**13**:2045-2056

[8] Barsotti S, Di Battista M, Venturini V, Della Rossa A, Mosca M. Management of digital ulcers in systemic sclerosis. Chronic Wound Care Management Research. 2019;**6**:9-18

[9] Chifflot H, Fautrel B, Sordet C, Chatelus E, Sibilia J. Incidence and prevalence of systemic sclerosis: A systematic literature review. Seminars in Arthritis and Rheumatism. 2008;**37**:223-235

[10] Castro S, Jimenez S. Biomarkers in systemic sclerosis. Biomarkers in Medicine. 2010;**4**(1):133-147

[11] Jerjen R, Nikpour M, Krieg T, Denton CP, Saracino AM. Systemic sclerosis in adults. Part I: Clinical features and pathogenesis. Journal of the American Academy of Dermatology. 2022;**87**(5):937-954. DOI: 10.1016/j.jaad.2021.10.065

[12] Snarskaya ES, Vasileva KD. Localized scleroderma: Actual insights and new biomarkers. International Journal of Dermatology. 2022;**61**(6):667-674. DOI: 10.1111/ijd.15811

[13] Rongioletti F, Ferreli C, Atzori L, Bottoni U, Soda G. Scleroderma with an update about clinico-pathological correlation. Giornale Italiano di Dermatologia e Venereologia. 2018;**153**(2):208-215. DOI: 10.23736/S0392-0488.18.05922-9

[14] Wenzel D, Haddadi NS, Afshari K, Richmond JM, Rashighi M. Upcoming treatments for morphea. Immunity Inflammation Diseases. 2021;**9**(4):1101-1145. DOI: 10.1002/iid3.475

[15] Guiducci S, Giacomelli R, Cerinic MM. Vascular complications of scleroderma. Autoimmunity Reviews. 2007;**6**(8):520-523. DOI: 10.1016/j.autrev.2006.12.006

[16] Gigante A, Leodori G, Pellicano C, Villa A, Rosato E. Assessment of kidney involvement in systemic sclerosis: From scleroderma renal crisis to subclinical renal vasculopathy. The American Journal of the Medical Sciences. 2022;**364**(5):529-537. DOI: 10.1016/j.amjms.2022.02.014

[17] Flavahan NA. New mechanism-based approaches to treating and evaluating the vasculopathy of scleroderma. Current Opinion in Rheumatology. 2021;**33**(6):471-479. DOI: 10.1097/BOR.0000000000000830

[18] Stochmal A, Czuwara J, Trojanowska M, Rudnicka L. Antinuclear antibodies in systemic sclerosis: An update. Clinical Reviews in Allergy and Immunology. 2020;**58**(1):40-51. DOI: 10.1007/s12016-018-8718-8

[19] Samuelsen S, Jørgensen CD, Mellins ED, Torok KS, Astakhova K. Detection of autoimmune antibodies in localized scleroderma by synthetic oligonucleotide antigens. PLoS One. 2018;**13**(4):e0195381. DOI: 10.1371/journal.pone.0195381

[20] Zhao M, Wu J, Wu H, Sawalha AH, Lu Q. Clinical treatment options in scleroderma: Recommendations and comprehensive review. Clinical Reviews in Allergy and Immunology. 2022;**62**(2):273-291. DOI: 10.1007/s12016-020-08831-4

[21] Distler O, Assassi S, Cottin V, Cutolo M, Danoff SK, Denton CP, et al. Predictors of progression in systemic sclerosis patients with interstitial lung disease. The European Respiratory Journal. 2020;**55**(5):1902026. DOI: 10.1183/13993003.02026-2019

[22] Showalter K, Hoffmann A, Rouleau G, Aaby D, Lee J, Richardson C, et al. Performance of forced vital capacity and lung diffusion cutpoints for associated radiographic interstitial lung disease in systemic sclerosis. Journal of Rheumatology. 2018;**45**(11):1572-1576. DOI: 10.3899/jrheum.171362

[23] Gur C, Wang SY, Sheban F, Zada M, Li B, Kharouf F, et al. LGR5 expressing skin fibroblasts define a major cellular hub perturbed in scleroderma. Cell. 2022;**185**(8):1373-1388.e20. DOI: 10.1016/j.cell.2022.03.011

[24] Hu M, Yao Z, Xu L, Peng M, Deng G, Liu L, et al. M2 macrophage polarization in systemic sclerosis fibrosis: Pathogenic mechanisms and therapeutic effects. Heliyon. 2023;**9**(5):e16206. DOI: 10.1016/j.heliyon.2023.e16206. PMID: 37234611; PMCID: PMC10208842

[25] Denton CP, Ong VH, Xu S, Chen-Harris H, Modrusan Z, Lafyatis R, et al. Therapeutic interleukin-6 blockade reverses transforming growth factor-beta pathway activation in dermal fibroblasts: Insights from the faSScinate clinical trial in systemic sclerosis. Annals of the Rheumatic Diseases. 2018;**77**(9):1362-1371

[26] Frerix M, Meier FM, Hermann W, Müller-Ladner U. Therapeutische Strategien im Frühstadium der systemischen Sklerose: Frühe Diagnose – frühe Symptome – frühe Probleme [Therapeutic management in early disease stages of systemic sclerosis: Early diagnosis – early symptoms – early problems]. Z Rheumatology. 2013;**72**(10):960-969. DOI: 10.1007/s00393-013-1270-2

[27] Andreasson K, Lillpers K, Wollheim F, Hesselstrand R. Systemisk skleros – en ovanlig men viktig diagnos i primärvården [Systemic sclerosis – a rare but important diagnosis in primary health care]. Lakartidningen. 2019;**26**:116

[28] Bellando-Randone S, Matucci-Cerinic M. Very early systemic sclerosis. Best Practice & Research. Clinical Rheumatology. 2019;**33**(4):101428. DOI: 10.1016/j.berh.2019.101428

[29] Matucci-Cerinic M, Allanore Y, Czirják L, Tyndall A, Müller-Ladner U, Denton C, et al. The challenge of early systemic sclerosis for the EULAR Scleroderma Trial and Research group (EUSTAR) community. It is time to cut the Gordian knot and develop a prevention or rescue strategy. Annals of the Rheumatic Diseases. 2009;**68**(9):1377-1380. DOI: 10.1136/ard.2008.106302

[30] Saito A, Horie M, Nagase T. TGF-β Signaling in lung health and disease. International Journal of Molecular Sciences. 2018;**19**(8):2460. DOI: 10.3390/ijms19082460

[31] Matarese G, Isola G, Anastasi GP, Favaloro A, Milardi D, Vermiglio G, et al. Immunohistochemical analysis of TGF-β1 and VEGF in gingival and periodontal tissues: A role of these biomarkers in the pathogenesis of scleroderma and periodontal disease. International Journal of Molecular Medicine. 2012;**30**(3):502-508. DOI: 10.3892/ijmm.2012.1024

[32] Yu JF, Jin YB, He J, An Y, Li ZG. Changes of serum Krebs von den Lungen-6 levels in interstitial lung disease associated with dermatomyositis and secondary Sjögren's syndrome: A case report. Beijing Da Xue Xue Bao Yi Xue Ban. 2017;**49**(5):910-914

[33] Benyamine A, Heim X, Resseguier N, Bertin D, Gomez C, Ebbo M, et al. Elevated serum Krebs von den Lungen-6 in systemic sclerosis: A marker of lung fibrosis and severity of the disease. Rheumatology International. 2018;**38**(5):813-819. DOI: 10.1007/s00296-018-3987-3

[34] Asano Y, Ihn H, Yamane K, et al. Clinical significance of surfactant protein D as a serum marker for evaluating pulmonary fibrosis in patients with systemic sclerosis. Arthritis and Rheumatism. 2001;**44**(6):1363-1369

[35] Hant F, Ludwicka-Bradley A, Wang H, et al. Surfactant protein D and KL-6 as serum biomarkers of interstitial lung disease in patients with scleroderma. The Journal of Rheumatology. 2009;**36**(4):773-780

[36] Khanna D, CJF L, Furst DE, et al. Tocilizumab in systemic sclerosis: A randomised, double-blind, placebo-controlled, phase 3 trial. Lancet Respiration Medicine. 2020;**8**(10):963-974. DOI: 10.1016/S2213-2600(20)30318-0. Erratum in: Lancet Respir Med. 2020 Oct;8(10):e75. Erratum in: Lancet Respir Med. 2021 Mar;9(3):e29

[37] Brown M, O'Reilly S. The immunopathogenesis of fibrosis in systemic sclerosis. Clinical Experimental Immunology. 2019;**195**(3):310-321. DOI: 10.1111/cei.13238

[38] De Lauretis A, Sestini P, Pantelidis P, et al. Serum interleukin 6 is predictive of early functional decline and mortality in interstitial lung disease associated with systemic sclerosis. The Journal of Rheumatology. 2013;**40**(4):435-446

[39] Wuttge D, Wildt M, Geborek P, Wollheim F, Scheja A, Akesson A. Serum IL-15 in patients with early systemic sclerosis: A potential novel marker of lung disease. Arthritis Research & Therapy. 2007;**9**(5):R85

[40] Asano Y, Stawski L, Hant F, et al. Endothelial Fli1 deficiency impairs vascular homeostasis: A role in scleroderma vasculopathy. The American Journal of Pathology. 2010;**176**:1983-1998

[41] Truchetet M, Brembilla N, Montanari E, Allanore Y, Chizzolini C. Increased frequency of circulating Th22 in addition to Th17 and Th2 lymphocytes in systemic sclerosis: Association with interstitial lung disease. Arthritis Research & Therapy. 2011;**13**(5):R166

[42] Mukherjee M, Mercurio V, Tedford R, et al. Right ventricular longitudinal strain is diminished in systemic sclerosis compared with idiopathic pulmonary arterial hypertension. The European Respiratory Journal. 2017;**50**:1701436

[43] Tardella M, Di Carlo M, Carotti M, Filippucci E, Grassi W, Salaffi F. Ultrasound B-lines in the evaluation of interstitial lung disease in patients with systemic sclerosis: Cut-off point definition for the presence of significant pulmonary fibrosis. Medicine (Baltimore). 2018;**97**:e0566

[44] Wu W, Jordan S, Becker M, et al. Prediction of progression of interstitial lung disease in patients with systemic sclerosis: The SPAR model. Annals of the Rheumatic Diseases. 2018;**77**:1326-1332

[45] Mohammadi A, Oshnoei S, Ghasemirad M. Comparison of a new, modified lung ultrasonography technique with high-resolution CT in the diagnosis of the alveolo-interstitial syndrome of systemic scleroderma. Medical Ultrasonography. 2014;**16**:27-31

[46] Wang Y, Gargani L, Barskova T, De F, Matucci-Cerinic M. Usefulness of lung ultrasound B-lines in connective tissue disease-associated interstitial lung disease: A literature review. Arthritis Research & Therapy. 2017;**19**:206

[47] Gargani L, Lionetti V, Di Cristofano C, Bevilacqua G, Recchia F, Picano E. Early detection of acute lung injury uncoupled to hypoxemia in pigs using ultrasound lung comets. Critical Care Medicine. 2007;**35**:2769-2774

[48] Doveri M, Frassi F, Consensi A, et al. Ultrasound lung comets: New echographic sign of lung interstitial fibrosis in systemic sclerosis. Reumatismo. 2008;**60**:180-184

[49] Barsotti S, Stagnaro C, d'Ascanio A, Della Rossa A. One year in review 2016: Systemic sclerosis. Clinical and Experimental Rheumatology. 34 Sep-Oct 2016;Suppl **100**(5):3-13. Epub 2016 Jul 18. PMID: 27463613

[50] Pinal Fernández I, Pallisa Núñez E, et al. Correlation of ultrasound B-lines with high-resolution computed tomography in antisynthetase syndrome. Clinical and Experimental Rheumatology. 2014;**32**:404-407

[51] Volpicelli G, Elbarbary M, Blaivas M, et al. International evidence-based recommendations for point-of-care lung ultrasound. Intensive Care Medicine. 2012;**38**:577-591

[52] Picano E, Frassi F, Agricola E, Gligorova S, Gargani L, Mottola G. Ultrasound lung comets: A clinically useful sign of extravascular lung water. Journal of the American Society of Echocardiography. 2006;**19**:356-363

[53] Diot E, Boissinot E, Asquier E, et al. Relationship between abnormalities on high-resolution CT and pulmonary function in systemic sclerosis. Chest. 1998;**114**:1623-1629

[54] Sperandeo M, Varriale A, Sperandeo G, Filabozzi P, Piattelli M, Carnevale V, et al. Transthoracic ultrasound in the evaluation of pulmonary fibrosis: Our experience. Ultrasound in Medicine & Biology. 2009;**35**:723-739

[55] Kim E, Lee K, Johkoh T, Kim T, Suh G, Kwon O, et al. Interstitial lung diseases associated with collagen vascular diseases: Radiologic and

histopathologic findings. Radiographics. 2002;**22**:S151-S165

[56] Bernstein E, Khanna D, Lederer D. Screening high-resolution computed tomography of the chest to detect interstitial lung disease in systemic sclerosis: A global survey of rheumatologists. Arthritis & Rhematology. 2018;**70**:971-972

[57] Coghlan JG, Pope J, Denton CP. Assessment of endpoints in pulmonary arterial hypertension associated with connective tissue disease. Current Opinion in Pulmonary Medicine. 2010;**16**(Suppl 1): S27-S34. DOI: 10.1097/01.mcp.0000370208.45756.e8

[58] Denton CP, Khanna D. Systemic sclerosis. Lancet. 2017;**390**(10103): 1685-1699. DOI: 10.1016/S0140-6736(17)30933-9

[59] Perelas A, Silver RM, Arrossi AV, Highland KB. Systemic sclerosis-associated interstitial lung disease. The Lancet Respiratory Medicine. 2020;**8**(3):304-320. DOI: 10.1016/S2213-2600(19)30480-1

[60] Choudhary SS, Choudhary S. Exercise testing in assessment and management of patients in clinical practice - present situation. Lung India. 2008;**25**(3):111-117. DOI: 10.4103/0970-2113.59592

[61] Balke B. A simple field test for the assessment of physical fitness. CARI Report. 1963;**63**:18

[62] Butland RJ, Pang J, Gross ER, et al. Two-, six, and 12-minute walking tests in respiratory disease. BMJ. 1982;**284**:1607-1608

[63] McGavin CR, Gupta SP, McHardy GJR. Twelve-minute walking test for assessing disability in chronic bronchitis. BMJ. 1976;**1**:822-823

[64] Sanges S, Giovannelli J, Sobanski V, et al. Factors associated with the 6-minute walk distance in patients with systemic sclerosis. Arthritis Research & Therapy. 2017;**19**(1):279. DOI: 10.1186/s13075-017-1489-4

[65] Vandecasteele E, Thevissen K, Melsens K, et al. Six-minute walk test in or out in evaluation of systemic sclerosis patients? Clinical and Experimental Rheumatology. 2017;**35**(Suppl. 106):S122-S129

[66] Pugnet G, Marjanovic Z, Deligny C, et al. Reproducibility and utility of the 6-min- ute walk test in systemic sclerosis. The Journal of Rheumatology. 2018;**45**:1273-1280

[67] Nguyenkim T, Maurer B, Suliman Y, Morsbach F, Distler O, Frauenfelder T. The impact of slice-reduced computed tomography on histogram-based densitometry assessment of lung fibrosis in patients with systemic sclerosis. Journal of Thoracic Disease. 2018;**10**:2142-2152

[68] Solway S, Brooks D, Lacasse Y, et al. A qualitative systematic overview of the measurement properties of functional walk tests used in the cardiorespiratory domain. Chest. 2001;**119**:256-270

[69] Enright PL, Mcburnie MA, Bittner V, Tracy RP, Mcnamara R, Arnold A, et al. The 6-min walk test: A quick measure of functional status in elderly adults. Chest. 2003;**123**(2):387-398

[70] Enright PL, Sherrill DL. Reference equations for the six-minute walk in healthy adults. American Journal of Respiratory and Critical Care Medicine. 1998;**158**(5 Pt 1):1384-1387

[71] Gibbons WJ, Fruchter N, Sloan S, Levy RD. Reference values for a multiple repetition 6-minute walk test in healthy

adults older than 20 years. Journal of Cardiopulmonary Rehabilitation. 2001;**21**(2):87-89

[72] Garin MC, Highland KB, Silver RM, Strange C. Limitations to the 6-minute walk test in interstitial lung disease and pulmonary hypertension in scleroderma. The Journal of Rheumatology. 2009;**36**(2):330-336. DOI: 10.3899/jrheum.080447

[73] Someya F, Mugii N, Oohata S. Factors relating to impaired stroke volume during the 6-minute walk test in patients with systemic sclerosis. Clinical Experimental in Rheumatology. 2016;**34**(5):152-156

[74] Vandecasteele E, Thevissen K, Melsens K, De Keyser F, De Pauw M, Deschepper E, et al. Six-minute walk test in or out in evaluation of systemic sclerosis patients? Clinical Experimental in Rheumatology. 2017;**106**(4):122-129

[75] Sanges S, Rice L, Tu L, Valenzi E, Cracowski JL, Montani D, et al. Biomarkers of haemodynamic severity of systemic sclerosis-associated pulmonary arterial hypertension by serum proteome analysis. Annals of the Rheumatic Diseases. Mar 2023;**82**(3):365-373. DOI: 10.1136/ard-2022-223237. Epub 2022 Dec 5. PMID: 36600187; PMCID: PMC9918672

Chapter 6

Important Considerations for Bone Health Management in Systemic Sclerosis Patients

Madeleine E. Frech, Ganiat Adeogun, Erin Chew, Tracy M. Frech and S. Bobo Tanner

Abstract

Bone health in systemic sclerosis (SSc) is an essential management consideration for rheumatologists caring for these patients. Screening for reduction in bone density includes a detailed health history, which includes SSc disease features such as intestinal malabsorption, patulous esophagus, and calcinosis. The established International Society for Clinical Densitometry (ISCD) guidelines provide an official position statement on important topics in skeletal assessment. Bone health laboratory testing are indicated in all SSc patients, especially if a low serum albumin or vitamin deficiencies are detected. Bone health treatment considerations include adequate weight bearing exercise, calcium, and vitamin D in all SSc patients. The key findings of this chapter is that SSc patients are at increased risk for low bone density and comorbidities may affect choice of treatment such as oral bisphosphonates in SSc patients with significant esophageal disease or renal impairment and osteoanabolic therapies in SSc patients with calcinosis are important.

Keywords: scleroderma, systemic sclerosis, osteoporosis, osteopenia, bone density

1. Introduction

Patients with systemic sclerosis (SSc, scleroderma) are reported to have a significant reduction in bone mass with an increased risk of vertebral fracture, especially with a longer disease duration [1, 2]. One meta-analysis published in 2020 evaluated 18 studies using pooled weighted mean difference (WMD) to estimate the mean difference in BMD between patients with SSc and controls showed that patients with SSc had significantly lower bone mineral density (BMD) than controls in the following categories: whole body (WMD − 0.07, 95% CI − 0.1 to − 0.04, $p < 0.00001$), lumbar spine (WMD − 0.08, 95% CI − 0.11 to − 0.05, $p < 0.00001$), femoral neck (WMD: −0.28, 95% CI: −0.46 to −0.10, $p = 0.002$), total hip (WMD − 0.10, 95% CI − 0.14 to − 0.06, $p < 0.00001$), and femoral trochanter (WMD − 0.06, 95% CI − 0.09 to − 0.03, $p < 0.0001$) [1]. While this meta-analysis did not find a significant difference in the risk of osteoporotic fracture between patients with SSc and controls (OR = 2.24, 95% CI 0.58 to 8.59, $p = 0.24$), the patients

IntechOpen

with SSc had an increased risk of vertebral fracture (OR 10.38, 95% CI 1.19 to 90.58, $p = 0.03$) [1]. In a subsequent meta-analysis, the pooled prevalence of osteoporosis in patients with SSc was 27% (95% CI, 24–31), with moderate heterogeneity ($I^2 = 61.6\%$) [2]. Meta-regression analysis was conducted to explore the sources of heterogeneity. This analysis of 22 studies identified significant risk factors for osteoporosis in SSc patients were age > 50 years (OR = 2.94, 95% CI, 1.52–5.68), menopause (OR = 3.90; 95% CI, 1.94–7.84), aging (MD = 8.40; 95% CI,6.10–10.71) and longer disease duration (MD = 4.78; 95% CI,1.83–7.73). However, female (OR = 1.45; 95% CI, 0.75–2.77), pulmonary arterial hypertension (OR = 0.50; 95% CI, 0.17–1.54), and diffuse cutaneous SSc (OR = 1.05; 95% CI, 0.75–1.48) were not significant risk factors for osteoporosis in SSc patients [2]. This data suggests osteoporosis is highly prevalent in patients with SSc, and similar in many countries, however a consensus approach on treatment of SSc osteoporosis is lacking. While these studies assessing epidemiology of osteoporosis in SSc are important, longitudinal data on treatment are lacking.

Early monitoring of bone mineral density in patients with SSc is recommended for the prevention of osteoporosis and fracture. However, treatment of low bone mineral density once detected can be a challenge to the treating physician. While treatment courses and monitoring of therapies are not within the scope of this review, SSc disease features such as intestinal malabsorption, patulous esophagus, and calcinosis are discussed as important considerations for bone health management in SSc patients.

2. Bone health screening

A bone health history must include consideration of age, sex, low body mass index, previous fragility fracture, parental history of hip fracture, glucocorticoid (GC) treatment, current smoking, and alcohol intake of 3 or more units daily to identify individuals at or above a 'fracture threshold' by the Fracture Risk Assessment Tool (FRAX). This fracture risk prediction tool was released in 2008 and provides country-specific algorithms to estimate the 10-year fracture risk using clinical and radiological data [3]. A dual energy X-ray absorptiometry (DXA) at the lumbar spine, total hip, and femoral neck for all patients is the gold standard for assessing bone mineral density (BMD) and is most often described as a T-score or Z-score, both of which are units of standard deviation (SD). The T-score describes the number of SDs by which the BMD in an individual differs from the mean value expected in young healthy individuals. The operational definition of osteoporosis is based on the T-score for BMD assessed at the femoral neck and is defined as a value for BMD 2.5 SD or more below the young female adult mean (T-score less than or equal to −2.5 SD) [4]. Functional status and fall frequency are not accounted for in the FRAX and are important considerations in SSc.

The International Society for Clinical Densitometry (ISCD) provides official position statements on important topics in skeletal assessment, through a rigorous, validated method for recommendations that are not accounted for in the current version of FRAX [5]. The ISCD includes recommendations for lumbar spine, total hip and one-third (33%) radius T-scores [6] in certain circumstances, such as severe obesity or hyperparathyroidism in post-menopausal women. Expert opinion suggests bone densitometry using DXA may underestimate fracture risk in younger SSc patients. Trabecular bone score (TBS) and vertebral fracture assessments (VFA) are novel tools that may offer additional information to improve fracture prediction in chronic inflammatory disease, and may have applicability to SSc [7–9]. TBS is an adjunctive software application on DXA machines that performs novel gray-level texture measurements on lumbar spine DXA images, capturing information relating to trabecular microarchitecture [10]. While TBS values were similar in a small cohort of SSc patients, systematic coupling of VFA with BMD allowed the diagnosis previously unknown asymptomatic vertebral fractures [11]. Other imaging methods have been used in chronic inflammatory disease to assess bone deficits and independently predict fracture risk, such as quantitative ultrasound or peripheral quantitative computed tomography, however, these approaches are not currently accepted as routine screening tests [12].

There are no specific guidelines for DXA in SSc, however the recommendations for individuals with rheumatoid arthritis (RA), a more common rheumatic disease, can provide some guidance, with a recommendation to screen all patients over age 50 [12]. Both high daily and cumulative glucocorticoid (GC) doses increase risk of fracture, particularly vertebral fracture, due to the greater effects of GCs on trabecular bone than on cortical bone. Steroids should be avoided in SSc due to scleroderma renal crisis risk. However, if a SSc patient has inflammatory features requiring low-dose glucocorticoids, greater or equal to 2.5 mg per day for 3 months or longer, BMD screening age should include anyone 40 years and older [13]. Screening frequency should be based on ongoing risk factors. Based on RA literature, BMD screening in 3 to 5-year intervals for SSc who have normal BMD, well-controlled disease, and are not taking GCs could be considered. Whereas whole body bone, fat and lean mass can also be measured using DXA, these measurements do not assist in the routine diagnosis or assessment of osteoporosis [14].

3. Laboratory assessment

The initial basic bone health laboratory testing should consist of complete blood count (CBC), serum calcium, phosphorus, creatinine with estimated glomerular filtration rate (eGFR), 24 h urinary calcium and creatinine excretion panel, hepatic function tests (including a gamma-glutamyl transferase, if the alkaline phosphatase is elevated), thyroid stimulating hormone, parathyroid hormone, and serum 25-OH-D [12]. If a decreased serum albumin is detected in the screening assessment, additional studies can include serum protein electrophoresis, quantitative immunoglobulins with serum free light chains, and stool alpha-1 antitrypsin [12, 15]. If malabsorption is suspected, hydrogen breath testing can be useful for the diagnosis of small intestinal bacterial overgrowth (SIBO) as many patients with this complication may suffer from nutritional deficiencies and osteoporosis. However, SIBO testing may not be readily available outside of academic medical centers. If vitamins (B12, D, A, and E) as well as minerals (iron and calcium) deficiencies are detected, in addition to empiric treatment for SIBO, celiac screening should be considered [16, 17]. Independent of diarrhea, low vitamin D and calcium levels may reflect malabsorption and can be a risk factor for secondary hyperparathyroidism and bone resorption [18]. The importance of understanding the gastrointestinal tract involvement in SSc is critical to a bone health management for not only calcium and vitamin D replacement, but also phosphorus and magnesium supplementation [4]. In the setting of renal disease, phosphate-lowering therapies may be indicated. The response of secondary osteoporosis to conventional anti-osteoporosis therapy may be inadequate if the underlying condition is unrecognized and untreated [8].

3.1 Treatment of osteoporosis

Bone mass reduction in SSc occurs with traditional risk factures such as age and menopausal status, but due to gastrointestinal tract disease may have additional risk factors as identified by history or laboratory assessment (**Figure 1**). Therefore, in addition to risk factor modification, the treatment of osteoporosis must include assessment for calcium and vitamin D, and consideration of medication interventions (**Table 1**).

3.2 Calcium and vitamin D

Confirmation of adequate calcium and vitamin D is an important step in osteoporosis management. Serum calcium levels are not an indication of nutritional calcium status. Validation of adequate calcium intake and absorption requires a 24-hour urine collection and analysis [19]. Laboratory "normal range reference intervals" for 24-hour calcium may vary by the race of the individual [20]. Recommendations

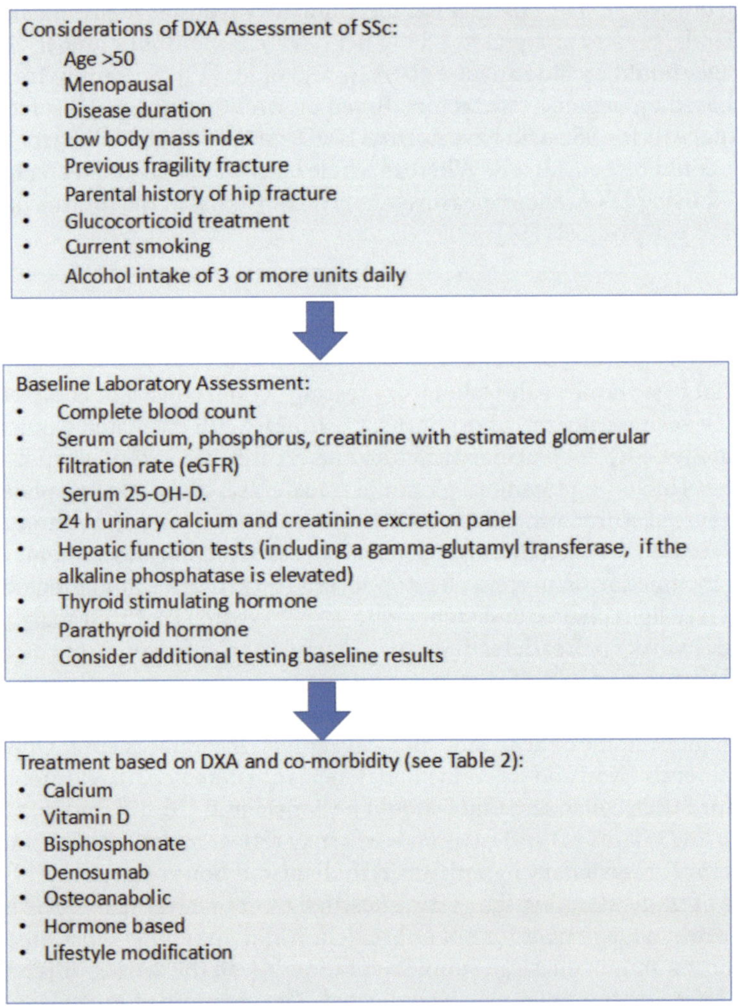

Figure 1.
Approach to bone health assessment in systemic sclerosis

Medication class	Important consideration of SSc disease features
Bisphosphonate	Consider if history of patulous esophagus, esophagitis, and reduced renal function.
Denosumab	Consider if history of erosive "RA-like" arthritis
Osteoanabolic	Consider if history of calcinosis
Hormone-based therapies	Consider if history of thrombosis

Table 1.
Medication class considerations.

should include a daily calcium intake of between 800 and 1200 mg and sufficient dietary protein, ideally achieved through dairy products [14]. Supplement use is recommended if adequate dietary intake is not achieved. Calcium supplement absorption and side effects may vary according to the calcium salt (e.g., calcium citrate vs. calcium carbonate or calcium formate). It is important to ask patients on calcium supplements about constipation, bloating, kidney stones, and possible vascular disease, which though not proven, is certainly a consideration in SSc [21]. As such, a dietary source rather than pill supplementation of calcium is preferred [22]. Supplementation with calcium alone does not reduce fracture risk, and vitamin D supplementation, rather than calcium, though controversial, may reduce falls risk in the elderly when combined with other prevention approaches [14, 23, 24].

Vitamin D replacement, 400–1000 IU per day, is generally recommended in patients receiving bone protective therapy and is proposed to not only have a beneficial effect on bone health, but may have a positive effect on the immune system in autoimmune disease [25, 26]. Lower vitamin D levels are reported in SSc with diffuse cutaneous disease when compared to the limited cutaneous subset [27]. The correct threshold for vitamin D replacement is debated due to differences in prior study designs, analysis, and randomized controlled trials. However, in RA the recommendation is to achieve 25-OH vitamin D level greater than 25 ng/ml to prevent hypocalcemia, especially in patients with chronic kidney disease receiving potent anti-resorptive drugs [12].

Calcinosis in SSc is associated with acro-osteolysis, digital ulceration, and osteoporosis, suggesting a link to severe vasculopathy [12]. Dystrophic soft-tissue calcification occurs in damaged or devitalized tissues in the presence of normal calcium/phosphorus metabolism and normal serum calcium and phosphorus levels [28]. Soft-tissue mineralization is a tightly regulated process relying on the activity of systemic and tissue-specific inhibitors and promoters of calcium precipitation. In SSc, this process is thought to be related to vascular hypoxia and in myositis-overlap disease related to release of calcium from mitochondria in damaged muscle cells [29]. The primary mineral component of calcinosis is hydroxyapatite in systemic sclerosis and carbonate apatite in dermatomyositis [29]. There is no published evidence related to calcium supplements and SSc calcinosis. However, radiologic scoring of calcinosis cutis offers an opportunity to objectively correlate this skin complication to reduction in BMD [30, 31].

3.3 Bisphosphonates

Bisphosphonates act by inhibiting osteoclast differentiation from osteoclast precursors. The oral bisphosphonates (alendronate, risedronate, ibandronate) may be used as initial treatments in most cases of osteoporosis, but potential gastrointestinal adverse effects are important considerations in SSc patients. Oral bisphosphonates are associated with mild gastrointestinal disturbances, and alendronate and pamidronate are associated with esophagitis, which is a concern in SSc patients with a patulous esophagus. Intravenous zoledronic acid has the highest probability of causing nausea and is associated with fever and bone and muscle pain that ameliorates or disappears after subsequent courses [32]. Osteonecrosis of the jaw has been described as an adverse effect of bisphosphonates and may be related to the class of bisphosphonate, differences in potency, and route of administration [14]. However, this potential adverse effect is often of concern to SSc patients with microstomia, in which dental procedures are challenging [33]. Bisphosphonates may have beneficial effects in a subgroup of calcinosis cutis patients [34]. Treatments should be reviewed after 3–5 years treatment with bisphosphonate, since a longer duration of bisphosphonates beyond 5 years has been associated with the risk of atypical femoral fracture. Fracture risk should be reassessed after a new fracture, regardless of when it occurs, because the risk of new fractures increases in patients who stop treatment [14].

3.4 Denosumab

The monoclonal antibody Denosumab is an inhibitor of receptor activator of nuclear factor-kB ligand (RANKL), which is necessary for osteoclast activation and survival. Prior trials comparing denosumab with other bisphosphonates in patients on GC led to greater spine and hip BMD gains, but there were no significant differences in fracture rates [35]. Trials have shown that denosumab decreases RA erosions [36]. Withdrawal of denosumab therapy is associated with a rebound in vertebral fracture rate, but adverse effects are in general non-significant [37]. Denosumab effect in SSc patients is not currently published.

3.5 Osteoanabolics

Teriparatide and abaloparatide are parathyroid hormone (PTH) analogs that stimulate osteoblast activity resulting in net bone formation [38]. The most common reported adverse events in patients treated with PTH analogs are nausea, pain in the limbs, headache and dizziness. Worsening of calcinosis cutis with teriparatide treatment in osteoporotic patients is reported in case reports [39, 40]. Romosozumab is a monoclonal antibody against sclerostin thereby stimulates osteoblasts with less concomitant activation of osteoclastic activity resulting in significant BMD gains and fracture prevention [41]. These treatments are considered in patients believed to be at very high risk for fracture, including those with a new or recent fracture or significant declining BMD on oral bisphosphonates or denosumab [42].

4. Hormone-based therapies

Raloxifene, a selective estrogen receptor modulator, stabilizes bone density and helps to prevent vertebral fractures in women, but it has not been shown to improve hip fracture rates [43].

American College of Rheumatology (ACR) 2017 Guideline for the Prevention and Treatment of Glucocorticoid-Induced Osteoporosis suggest it as a treatment option only for postmenopausal women with contraindications to other bone health agents and without thromboembolic risk [13]. Bazedoxifene is a third-generation selective estrogen receptor modulator (SERM) in the US was approved as combination drug along with conjugated estrogens to prevent post-menopausal osteoporosis achieves small but significant increases in the bone mineral density of the lumbar spine but not the total hip [44]. However, in pre-clinical models SERM-class drugs could treat SSc fibrosis [45].

Hypogonadism is a risk factor for osteoporosis. Testosterone treatment may be indicated in men with documented symptomatic androgen deficiency as it has been found to improve BMD but should not be used alone as an osteoporosis agent because there is no long-term anti-fracture efficacy data [46].

5. Lifestyle modification

Patients with SSc should be counseled on tobacco cessation, healthy diet, alcohol reduction, and weight-bearing exercise, especially if they have a reduction on BMD. Poor dietary habits, including high intake of sugar-sweetened beverages, are associated with hyperglycemia can decrease osteoblast proliferation and increase osteoclast activation [47]. A nutritionist is a critical partner on a SSc patient's team of providers, especially in SSc patients with low BMD [48, 49]. Formal exercise programs are recommended for SSc patients, with a focus on balance and fall prevention [50].

6. Conclusion

Bone health screening is a critical aspect of SSc patient care. However, SSc patients have disease features that are worth considering (**Figure 1**) [51]. In addition to referral for DXA, screening laboratories are critical to understand potential gastrointestinal and renal involvement that influence treatment decisions. Esophageal disease may limit bisphosphonate compliance, and denosumab is a reasonable choice in SSc patients. While the presence of calcinosis cutis should not limit calcium and vitamin D replacement, the use of PTH analogs may cause a worsening of lesions. SERM may have a beneficial anti-fibrotic effect but require further study and should be balanced against possible thromboembolic risk in these patients with vasculopathy. Healthy diet and weight-bearing exercise should be encouraged by the treating rheumatologist regardless of bone health status, but these become a critical aspect of the care plan when osteoporosis is diagnosed.

Disclosures

None.

Key points

- Bone health assessment, including medical history, screening laboratories, and dual energy X-ray absorptiometry, is a critical aspect of SSc patient care.

- Treatment of low bone mineral density once detected can be a challenge and the treating physician should avoid oral bisphosphonates in SSc patients with significant esophageal disease or renal impairment and osteoanabolic therapies in SSc patients with calcinosis.

Author details

Madeleine E. Frech[1*], Ganiat Adeogun[2], Erin Chew[2], Tracy M. Frech[2] and S. Bobo Tanner[2]

1 University of Notre Dame, South Bend, IN, USA

2 Department of Internal Medicine, Division of Rheumatology and Immunology, Vanderbilt University Medical Center, Nashville, TN, USA

*Address all correspondence to: mfrech2@nd.edu

References

[1] Chen J, Lei L, Pan J, Zhao C. A meta-analysis of fracture risk and bone mineral density in patients with systemic sclerosis. Clinical Rheumatology. 2020;**39**:1181-1189. DOI: 10.1007/s10067-019-04847-0

[2] Tu X et al. High prevalence and risk factors for osteoporosis in 1839 patients with systemic sclerosis: A systematic review and meta-analysis. Clinical Rheumatology. 2022;**42**(4):1087-1099. DOI: 10.1007/s10067-022-06460-0

[3] Kanis JA, Johnell O, Oden A, Johansson H, McCloskey E. FRAX and the assessment of fracture probability in men and women from the UK. Osteoporosis International. 2008;**19**:385-397. DOI: 10.1007/s00198-007-0543-5

[4] Rondanelli M et al. An update on magnesium and bone health. Biometals. 2021;**34**:715-736. DOI: 10.1007/s10534-021-00305-0

[5] Densitometry IS. Adult Official Positions of the ISCD. ISCD; 2019. Available from: https://iscd.org/wp-content/uploads/2021/09/2019-Official-Positions-Adult-1.pdf

[6] Arceo-Mendoza RM, Camacho PM. Postmenopausal Osteoporosis: Latest Guidelines. Endocrinology and Metabolism Clinics of North America. 2021;**50**:167-178. DOI: 10.1016/j.ecl.2021.03.009

[7] Akrapovic Olic I, Radic M. Comment on "a meta-analysis of fracture risk and bone mineral density in patients with systemic sclerosis". Clinical Rheumatology. 2020;**39**:2243-2244. DOI: 10.1007/s10067-020-05098-0

[8] Ebeling PR et al. Secondary osteoporosis. Endocrine Reviews. 2022;**43**:240-313. DOI: 10.1210/endrev/bnab028

[9] Shuhart CR et al. Executive summary of the 2019 ISCD position development conference on monitoring treatment, DXA cross-calibration and least significant change, spinal cord injury, Peri-prosthetic and orthopedic bone health, transgender medicine, and pediatrics. Journal of Clinical Densitometry. 2019;**22**:453-471. DOI: 10.1016/j.jocd.2019.07.001

[10] Silva BC et al. Trabecular bone score: A noninvasive analytical method based upon the DXA image. Journal of Bone and Mineral Research. 2014;**29**:518-530. DOI: 10.1002/jbmr.2176

[11] Lescoat A et al. Bone mineral density and trabecular bone score assessment in systemic sclerosis: A cross-sectional study. Joint, Bone, Spine. 2021;**88**:105214. DOI: 10.1016/j.jbspin.2021.105214

[12] Wysham KD, Baker JF, Narla R. Osteoporosis evaluation and treatment recommendations in rheumatoid arthritis. Best Practice & Research. Clinical Rheumatology. 2022;**36**:101757. DOI: 10.1016/j.berh.2022.101757

[13] Buckley L et al. 2017 American College of Rheumatology Guideline for the prevention and treatment of glucocorticoid-induced osteoporosis. Arthritis & Rhematology. 2017;**69**:1521-1537. DOI: 10.1002/art.40137

[14] Kanis JA et al. European guidance for the diagnosis and management of osteoporosis in postmenopausal women. Osteoporosis International. 2019;**30**:3-44. DOI: 10.1007/s00198-018-4704-5

[15] Lewiecki EM. Evaluating patients for secondary causes of osteoporosis.

Current Osteoporosis Reports. 2022;**20**:1-12. DOI: 10.1007/s11914-022-00717-y

[16] Losurdo G et al. The influence of small intestinal bacterial overgrowth in digestive and extra-intestinal disorders. International Journal of Molecular Sciences. 2020;**21**:3531. DOI: 10.3390/ijms21103531

[17] Bartoloni E et al. Celiac disease prevalence is increased in primary Sjogren's syndrome and diffuse systemic sclerosis: Lessons from a large multi-Center study. Journal of Clinical Medicine. 2019;**8**:540. DOI: 10.3390/jcm8040540

[18] Braun-Moscovici Y et al. Vitamin D, parathyroid hormone, and acroosteolysis in systemic sclerosis. The Journal of Rheumatology. 2008;**35**:2201-2205. DOI: 10.3899/jrheum.071171

[19] Blaine J, Chonchol M, Levi M. Renal control of calcium, phosphate, and magnesium homeostasis. Clinical Journal of the American Society of Nephrology. 2015;**10**:1257-1272. DOI: 10.2215/CJN.09750913

[20] Smith LM, Gallagher JC. Reference range for 24-h urine calcium, calcium/creatinine ratio, and correlations with calcium absorption and serum vitamin D metabolites in normal women. Osteoporosis International. 2021;**32**:539-547. DOI: 10.1007/s00198-020-05615-6

[21] Reid IR, Bolland MJ. Controversies in medicine: The role of calcium and vitamin D supplements in adults. The Medical Journal of Australia. 2019;**211**:468-473. DOI: 10.5694/mja2.50393

[22] Reid IR, Bristow SM, Bolland MJ. Calcium supplements: Benefits and risks. Journal of Internal Medicine. 2015;**278**:354-368. DOI: 10.1111/joim.12394

[23] Appel LJ et al. The effects of four doses of vitamin D supplements on falls in older adults: A response-adaptive, randomized clinical trial. Annals of Internal Medicine. 2021;**174**:145-156. DOI: 10.7326/M20-3812

[24] Pfortmueller CA, Lindner G, Exadaktylos AK. Reducing fall risk in the elderly: Risk factors and fall prevention, a systematic review. Minerva Medica. 2014;**105**:275-281

[25] Rosen Y, Daich J, Soliman I, Brathwaite E, Shoenfeld Y. Vitamin D and autoimmunity. Scandinavian Journal of Rheumatology. 2016;**45**:439-447. DOI: 10.3109/03009742.2016.1151072

[26] Macdonald HM et al. 25-Hydroxyvitamin D threshold for the effects of vitamin D supplements on bone density: Secondary analysis of a randomized controlled trial. Journal of Bone and Mineral Research. 2018;**33**:1464-1469. DOI: 10.1002/jbmr.3442

[27] An L, Sun MH, Chen F, Li JR. Vitamin D levels in systemic sclerosis patients: A meta-analysis. Drug Design, Development and Therapy. 2017;**11**:3119-3125. DOI: 10.2147/DDDT.S144860

[28] Boulman N, Slobodin G, Rozenbaum M, Rosner I. Calcinosis in rheumatic diseases. Seminars in Arthritis and Rheumatism. 2005;**34**:805-812. DOI: 10.1016/j.semarthrit.2005.01.016

[29] Valenzuela A, Chung L. Subcutaneous calcinosis: Is it different between systemic sclerosis and dermatomyositis? Journal of Scleroderma and Related Disorders. 2022;**7**:7-23. DOI: 10.1177/23971983211053245

[30] Valenzuela A et al. Change in calcinosis over 1 year using the scleroderma clinical trials consortium

radiologic scoring system for calcinosis of the hands in patients with systemic sclerosis. Seminars in Arthritis and Rheumatism. 2022;**53**:151980. DOI: 10.1016/j.semarthrit.2022.151980

[31] Fauny M et al. Relationship between ectopic calcifications and bone fragility depicted on computed tomography scan in 70 patients with systemic sclerosis. Journal of Scleroderma and Related Disorders. 2022;**7**:224-233. DOI: 10.1177/23971983221104415

[32] Tadrous M et al. Comparative gastrointestinal safety of bisphosphonates in primary osteoporosis: A network meta-analysis. Osteoporosis International. 2014;**25**:1225-1235. DOI: 10.1007/s00198-013-2576-2

[33] Veale BJ, Jablonski RY, Frech TM, Pauling JD. Orofacial manifestations of systemic sclerosis. British Dental Journal. 2016;**221**:305-310. DOI: 10.1038/sj.bdj.2016.678

[34] Rauch L, Hein R, Biedermann T, Eyerich K, Lauffer F. Bisphosphonates for the treatment of calcinosis cutis-a retrospective single-Center study. Biomedicine. 2021;**9**:1698. DOI: 10.3390/biomedicines9111698

[35] Saag KG et al. Denosumab versus Risedronate in glucocorticoid-induced osteoporosis: Final results of a twenty-four-month randomized, double-blind, double-dummy trial. Arthritis & Rhematology. 2019;**71**:1174-1184. DOI: 10.1002/art.40874

[36] Takeuchi T et al. Effects of the anti-RANKL antibody denosumab on joint structural damage in patients with rheumatoid arthritis treated with conventional synthetic disease-modifying antirheumatic drugs (DESIRABLE study): A randomised, double-blind, placebo-controlled phase 3 trial. Annals of the Rheumatic Diseases. 2019;**78**:899-907. DOI: 10.1136/annrheumdis-2018-214827

[37] von Keyserlingk C et al. Clinical efficacy and safety of denosumab in postmenopausal women with low bone mineral density and osteoporosis: A meta-analysis. Seminars in Arthritis and Rheumatism. 2011;**41**:178-186. DOI: 10.1016/j.semarthrit.2011.03.005

[38] Sobh MM et al. Secondary osteoporosis and metabolic bone diseases. Journal of Clinical Medicine. 2022;**11**:2382. DOI: 10.3390/jcm11092382

[39] Echeverri AF et al. Worsening of calcinosis cutis with teriparatide treatment in two osteoporotic patients. The British Journal of Dermatology. 2016;**175**:1049-1051. DOI: 10.1111/bjd.14550

[40] Htet TD, Eisman JA, Elder GJ, Center JR. Worsening of soft tissue dystrophic calcification in an osteoporotic patient treated with teriparatide. Osteoporosis International. 2018;**29**:517-518. DOI: 10.1007/s00198-017-4330-7

[41] Singh S et al. A systematic review and meta-analysis of efficacy and safety of Romosozumab in postmenopausal osteoporosis. Osteoporosis International. 2022;**33**:1-12. DOI: 10.1007/s00198-021-06095-y

[42] Taylor AD, Saag KG. Anabolics in the management of glucocorticoid-induced osteoporosis: An evidence-based review of long-term safety, efficacy and place in therapy. Core Evidence. 2019;**14**:41-50. DOI: 10.2147/CE.S172820

[43] Ettinger B et al. Reduction of vertebral fracture risk in postmenopausal women with osteoporosis treated

with raloxifene: Results from a 3-year randomized clinical trial. Multiple outcomes of Raloxifene evaluation (MORE) investigators. JAMA. 1999;**282**:637-645. DOI: 10.1001/jama.282.7.637

[44] Yavropoulou MP, Makras P, Anastasilakis AD. Bazedoxifene for the treatment of osteoporosis. Expert Opinion on Pharmacotherapy. 2019;**20**:1201-1210. DOI: 10.1080/14656566.2019.1615882

[45] Kim Y, Nam Y, Rim YA, Ju JH. Anti-fibrotic effect of a selective estrogen receptor modulator in systemic sclerosis. Stem Cell Research & Therapy. 2022;**13**:303. DOI: 10.1186/s13287-022-02987-w

[46] Snyder PJ et al. Effect of testosterone treatment on volumetric bone density and strength in older men with low testosterone: A controlled clinical trial. JAMA Internal Medicine. 2017;**177**:471-479. DOI: 10.1001/jamainternmed.2016.9539

[47] Handel MN, Heitmann BL, Abrahamsen B. Nutrient and food intakes in early life and risk of childhood fractures: A systematic review and meta-analysis. The American Journal of Clinical Nutrition. 2015;**102**:1182-1195. DOI: 10.3945/ajcn.115.108456

[48] Allred D et al. Chronic multiorgan rare disease: The role of the nurse practitioner as a leader of the healthcare team. The Journal of Medical Practice Management. 2017;**32**:413-416

[49] Paolino S et al. Nutritional status and bone microarchitecture in a cohort of systemic sclerosis patients. Nutrients. 2020;**12**:1632. DOI: 10.3390/nu12061632

[50] Pettersson H et al. Exercise as a multi-modal disease-modifying medicine in systemic sclerosis: An introduction by the global fellowship on rehabilitation and exercise in systemic sclerosis (G-FoRSS). Best Practice & Research. Clinical Rheumatology. 2021;**35**:101695. DOI: 10.1016/j.berh.2021.101695

[51] Khosla S, Hofbauer LC. Osteoporosis treatment: Recent developments and ongoing challenges. The Lancet Diabetes and Endocrinology. 2017;**5**:898-907. DOI: 10.1016/S2213-8587(17)30188-2

Chapter 7

Skeletal Muscle Involvement in Systemic Sclerosis

Anja Srpčič, Felicita Urzi, Sanja Markez, Sergej Pirkmajer, Neža Brezovec, Katja Lakota and Katja Perdan Pirkmajer

Abstract

Systemic sclerosis (SSc) is a systemic autoimmune connective tissue disease with great clinical and pathogenetic heterogeneity. Although skin is the most visible organ affected, skeletal muscles are affected in up to 96% of SSc patients and this is associated with a worse clinical outcome including increased mortality. Muscle involvement varies from patients experiencing myalgias, fibrosing myopathy to overlaps of SSc and myositis, a condition referred to as scleromyositis. In SSc muscle biopsies, muscular fibrosis, inflammation, microangiopathy and atrophy are observed, which is consistent with most prominent SSc pathophysiologic processes. The damage and fibrosis of the muscle tissue and the reduced ability of the body to build and repair muscle lead to a loss of muscle mass and strength. Studies show that patients with SSc have a higher prevalence of myopenia than the general population, but the exact cause is not yet fully understood. Partially, this phenomenon could be attributed to the disrupted activity of fibro-adipogenic progenitors, driven by alterations in the skeletal muscle microenvironment of SSc patients. These changes are also reflected in shifts in myokine secretion.

Keywords: skeletal muscle, autoimmune myositis, systemic sclerosis, scleromyositis, myopathy, myopenia, myokines, fibro-adipogenic progenitors

1. Introduction

Systemic sclerosis (SSc) is an autoimmune connective tissue disease that most commonly occurs between 40 and 60 years of age [1] and affects women more often than men; however, male patients tend to have more severe disease [2].

Patients are clinically divided into limited cutaneous (lcSSc) and diffuse cutaneous (dcSSc) subsets based on the extent of skin involvement. The dcSSc subtype typically has a worse prognosis and more common development of joint contractures, skeletal myopathy, kidney disease, interstitial lung disease and heart involvement, while in lcSSc, digital ischemia, oesophageal disease, pulmonary arterial hypertension and malabsorption occur more commonly. SSc-specific anti-topoisomerase I autoantibodies are more prevalent in dcSSc, while anti-centromere antibodies are more prevalent in lcSSc [3].

IntechOpen

While muscle involvement is not the most life-threatening manifestation of SSc, musculoskeletal impairments are one of the main factors for physical disabilities that affect the ability to perform activities of daily living and can have a significant impact on patients' quality of life [4, 5]. It is important to stress that patients with myopathy also have more severe disease and decreased survival [6–9].

2. Characteristics of muscle involvement in SSc

Muscle involvement in SSc can present itself in a wide range of pathologies, from indolent subclinical myopathy that manifests as a mild muscle enzyme-level elevation, to aggressive inflammation as in idiopathic inflammatory myopathy. Sometimes it can present itself in a similar manner to other SSc organ involvements in the form of fibrosing myopathy without any existing evidence of inflammation [10].

The estimated prevalence of muscle involvement in SSc ranges widely from 5 to 96%. The variability in data reflects the lack of a formal definition of muscle involvement, which can include muscle weakness, abnormal muscle enzymes, abnormal electromyography (EMG) or abnormal biopsy of skeletal muscle [6]. Risk factors associated with myopathy are male gender, diffuse cutaneous SSc, shorter disease duration and higher modified Rodnan skin score [11].

2.1 Clinical features

Myalgia, muscle weakness and tenderness are being most frequently reported by patients, myalgia by 11 to 56% and muscle weakness by 23 to 60% of SSc patients. Objective muscle weakness detected on physical examination was present in 9 to 83% of cases. Patients generally present with symmetrical proximal upper and lower limb weaknesses. It is suggested that extra muscular involvement, such as skin thickening, interstitial lung disease, pulmonary arterial hypertension and anaemia, can also contribute to exercise limitation in SSc patients [10].

2.2 Laboratory findings

SSc patients with suspected myopathy should be tested for serum levels of muscle enzymes, creatine kinase (CK) and aldolase. Serum CK and aldolase elevation is reported in 6 to 47% and in 11 to 75% of SSc patients, respectively [8]. In the European Scleroderma Trials and Research group (EUSTAR) cohort, a substantial number of patients had muscle weakness, but not all of them had simultaneous CK elevation; 22.8% of patients with lcSSc and 37.1% of patients with dcSSc had muscle weakness, while 4.4 and 11.3% had elevated CK, respectively [12]. CK can also be elevated in myocarditis, where measurement of isoenzymes and serum troponin can be helpful in identifying CK origin [8]. All patients with SSc and suspicion of muscle involvement should also have their thyroid function tested. SSc patients can have specific autoantibodies, which can predict the clinical phenotype, and in patients with SSc-myositis overlap anti-Ku, anti-U1RNP and anti-PM-Scl are most prevalent among autoantibodies [13].

2.3 Electromyography

Laboratory markers can sometimes be unreliable; thus, electromyography (EMG) can be helpful to define the cause of muscle weakness and/or elevated levels of muscle enzymes. EMG was found to be abnormal in 11 to 92% of SSc patients. It is usually altered similar to EMG performed in patients with idiopathic inflammatory myopathies, as myopathic patterns are more frequently demonstrated in proximal than distal muscles [14].

2.4 Magnetic resonance imaging

Magnetic resonance imaging (MRI) can be helpful in determining the aetiology of muscle weakness in SSc patients and can help to identify an appropriate site for muscle biopsy. Muscle oedema is the most commonly reported finding on MRI, and changes such as fatty replacement of muscle tissue on T1 sequences can suggest chronic and irreversible muscle damage [14].

2.5 Muscle biopsy

Muscle biopsy in SSc patients can be helpful if the clinical picture is not clear. The histopathologic features are heterogeneous. According to the European Neuromuscular Centre (ENMC), there are four histopathologic categories of myopathy: polymyositis, dermatomyositis, necrotizing myopathy and non-specific myositis. In one study of 42 patients with SSc and muscle weakness, the most common histopathologic categories were non-specific myositis (35.7%) and necrotizing myopathy (21.4%). This study also showed that higher CK values were associated with inflammation and necrosis [14]. Another study demonstrated that fibrosis (81%) and microangiopathy (92%) are the main histopathologic hallmarks of SSc-related myopathy [15]. Therefore, histopathologic findings allow us to identify patients with predominant features related to inflammation and patients with features suggestive of fibrosis, which may be helpful when considering appropriate treatment.

2.6 Nailfold capillaroscopy

Studies have shown that muscle involvement was observed in 12 to 50% of SSc patients with advanced microvascular damage assessed with nailfold videocapillaroscopy (NVC) [16–18]. Patients with SSc exhibiting late NVC patterns were found to have decreased whole-body lean and fat mass compared to those with early and active NVC patterns [17]. The decrease in lean mass was more noticeable in the upper limbs, potentially indicating muscle wasting or loss of muscle mass in those areas [17]. It was observed that SSc patients with late NVC pattern had a significantly higher prevalence of low skeletal muscle index (43.75%), while in patients with early (9.1%) and active (12.5%) NVC patterns, the prevalence of a low skeletal muscle index was lower [16].

2.7 Skeletal muscle damage patterns in SSc

Muscle involvement in SSc can present in two major histopathological patterns distinguished by the predominating pathological process in skeletal muscle tissue. In one, fibrosis prevails, while in the other, inflammation is more pronounced (**Figure 1**).

2.8 Fibrosing myopathy

SSc patients with muscle weakness and fibrosing myopathy (fibrosis predominance on muscle biopsy) represent a subset of patients that tend to have dcSSc. They have

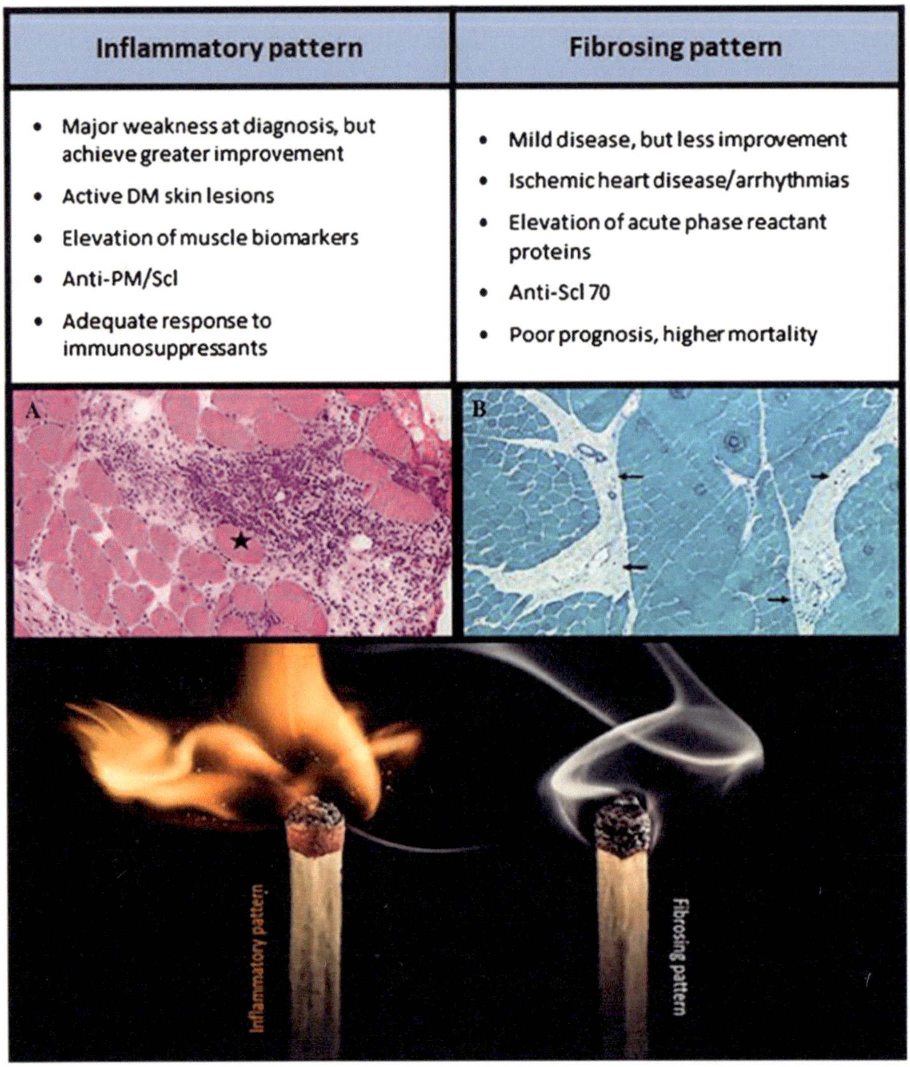

Figure 1.
Differences between inflammatory and fibrosing patterns of muscle involvement [19].

lower values of muscle enzymes (CK, aldolase), more prevalent non-irritable myopathy on EMG and higher mortality rates compared to SSc patients with muscle weakness and a muscle biopsy showing an inflammatory myopathy. The presence of anti-Scl-70 and anti-U3-RNP autoantibodies was detected more frequently in patients with fibrosing myopathy [20]. Patients with fibrosing myopathy show less therapeutic response and thus have a worse prognosis.

2.9 Scleromyositis

SSc and autoimmune myositis (AIM) are classic connective tissue diseases. We usually have specific diagnostic and/or classification criteria for these diseases, but sometimes a patient fulfils criteria for two different diseases. Scleromyositis, or SSc associated with myositis, is one of the best known and recognised overlap syndromes. Scleromyositis patients fulfil the criteria for SSc and AIM, have clinical features of both diseases and most of them also have specific immunological markers [8, 19]. Among myositis-associated autoantibodies, which are generally characteristic for patients with overlap myositis, anti-PM/Scl, anti-Ku, anti-U1RNP and anti-U3RNP are most common in SSc/AIM overlap. In a few patients, anti-RuvBL1/2 and anti-SMN autoantibodies have been reported (**Figure 2**). Despite the large panel of recognised autoantibodies, about half of SSc/AIM overlap patients are seronegative, meaning no currently known SSc-related autoantibodies can be detected in their serum samples [21]. Subsets of SSc/AIM overlap patients with different autoantibodies differ in the age of disease onset, response to treatment, risk of interstitial lung disease and survival [8].

Research studies indicate that muscle weakness, which is typically symmetrical, proximal, bilateral and more pronounced in the upper limbs, was observed in 13 to 100% of patients with scleromyositis. In addition, 21 to 88% of scleromyositis patients reported myalgias [8]. Other typical symptoms of scleromyositis include Raynaud's phenomenon occurring in approximately 81% of scleromyositis patients [22], and head dropping or camptocormia due to axial muscle weakness, which occurs in approximately one third of patients with SSc/AIM overlap [8].

Due to the systemic nature of the SSc/AIM disease, extramuscular symptoms are common (**Figure 3**), with approximately 33% of patients suffering from impaired forced vital capacity, 25% from dysphagia and 20% from cardiac involvement [22]. The higher frequency of extramuscular complications is a plausible explanation for the higher mortality among SSc/AIM overlap patients compared to SSc patients with no muscular involvement [8, 23]. The cumulative 5- and 10-year survival from diagnosis for SSc/AIM overlap patients is 82 and 68%, respectively, compared to 93 and 87% for SSc patients with no muscular involvement (**Figure 2**) [23]. In both, the most common cause of death is pulmonary complications, followed by cardiac complications, scleroderma renal crisis and gastrointestinal involvement [8]. Compared to SSc patients, SSc/AIM overlap patients have a higher risk of interstitial lung disease, one of the leading death-causing complications, and scleroderma renal crisis, which could be explained by the more frequent use of corticosteroids among SSc/AIM patients [8, 24].

A scoping review of 77 studies that included 559 muscle biopsies from SSc patients with myositis reported upregulation of sarcolemmal major histocompatibility

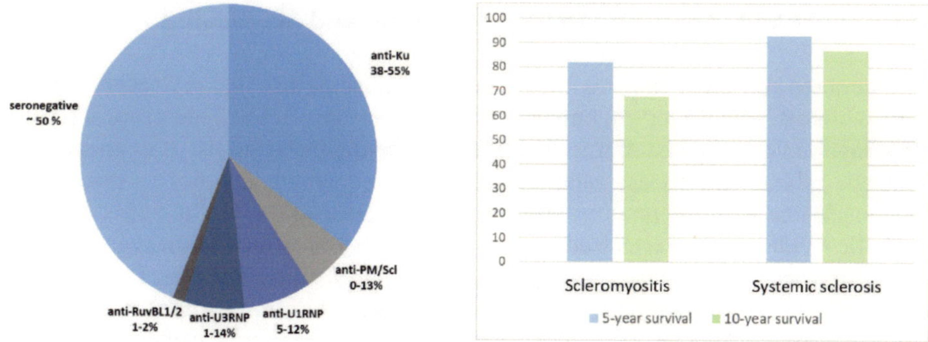

Figure 2.
Presence of autoantibodies in scleromyositis and survival in SSc and SSc/AIM overlap.

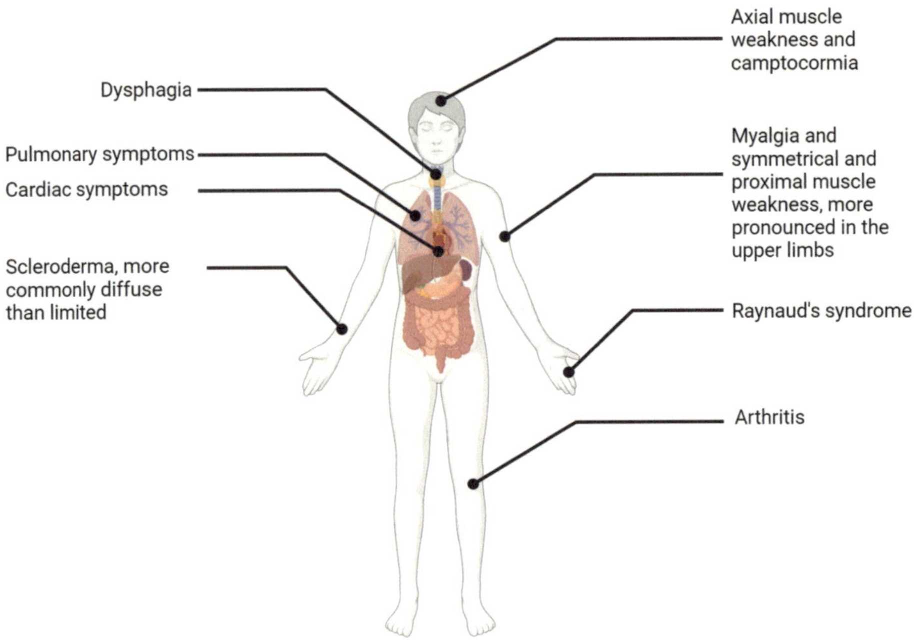

Figure 3.
Symptoms of scleromyositis.

complex class I (MHC-I) proteins (72%), inflammatory infiltrates (57%) that were predominantly T cell and present in endomysium, perimysium and perivascularly, muscle fibre necrosis (56%), myofibre atrophy (48%), regenerative fibres (41%), fibrosis (35%), neurogenic features (23%) and mitochondrial abnormalities (8%) [8, 25]. Vasculopathy and endomysial fibrosis, each present in approximately 33% of SSc/AIM overlap patients, may be the histopathological features suitable to distinguish SSc/AIM overlap from other forms of autoimmune myositis, which is consistent with the fact that vasculopathy and fibrosis are the two main features of SSc pathophysiology, along with immune dysfunction, a common feature with other AIM subgroups [25, 26]. These findings underscore the complex nature of muscle involvement in SSc, resulting from the interplay of vasculopathy, connective tissue and neurogenic changes, immune activation, and other factors.

3. Myopenia and sarcopenia in SSc: Screening and diagnosing

Sarcopenia and myopenia are impairments of musculature that may overlap in features but differ in underlying mechanisms and severity. It has been proposed to define myopenia as the loss of muscle mass in cachexia to distinguish it from sarcopenia, age-related and disease-related muscle wasting, which includes decrease in both muscle quantity and quality (strength and function) [27]. Cachexia is a complex metabolic syndrome characterised by the progressive loss of muscle mass and adipose tissue, often accompanied by systemic inflammation, insulin resistance and increased muscle protein breakdown [28], leading to progressive functional impairment [27]. Although malnutrition can occur in both cachexia and sarcopenia, cachexia is typically associated with a more pronounced and severe degree of malnutrition due to the underlying systemic disease and inflammatory state (**Figure 4**) [29].

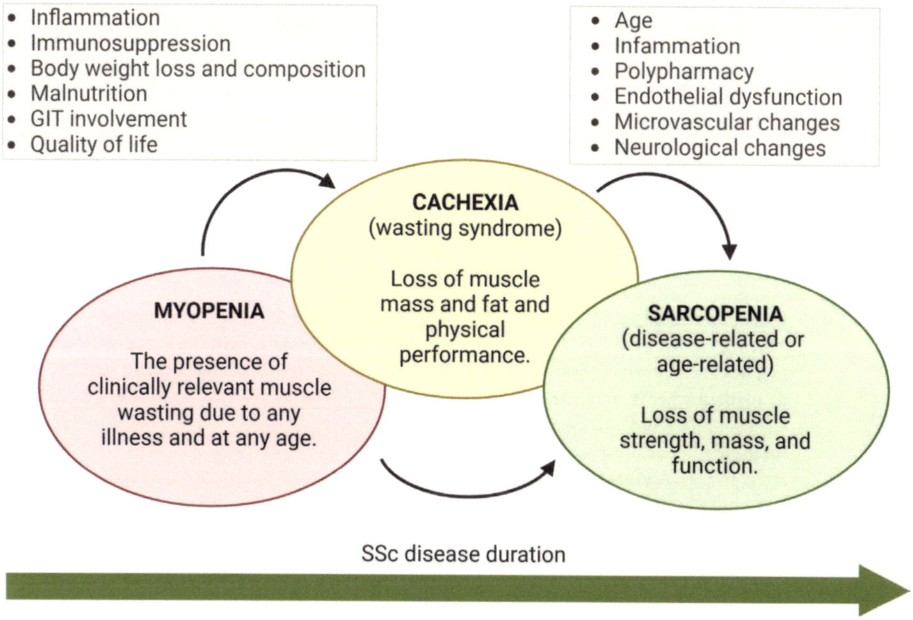

Figure 4.
Development of muscle loss in chronic disease.

Sarcopenia is recognised as a muscle disease with the ICD-10-CM (M62.84) code [30]. It occurs with ageing, inactivity, and/or disease, and increases the risk of falls, disability, and mortality. Over the past decade, many aspects of sarcopenia have been studied, and the definition and diagnostic criteria for sarcopenia have evolved. Originally, sarcopenia was described as an age-related decrease in lean body mass [31]; however, recently the definition and guidelines for the diagnosis of sarcopenia were prepared by the European Working Group on Sarcopenia in Older People (EWGSOP2) (**Table 1**) [33] requiring decreased muscle quantity or quality must be detected for diagnosis. In particular, the finding of low muscle strength is used as the primary parameter of sarcopenia. Muscle quality, defined as strength and/or power per unit of muscle mass, is an emerging biomarker that relates skeletal muscle structure to function [33, 37–39]. Muscle quality characteristics include factors such as structural changes in the neuromuscular system with loss of skeletal muscle contractile units, remodelling of fibre types and motor units, decreased muscle regenerative capacity, fat infiltration and mitochondrial dysfunction [40–42].

Impaired muscle function together with fatigue, and disability due to other SSc symptoms (such as skin fibrosis and nutrition issues) and chronic inflammation can lead to myopenia. Overall, the results of the studies show that the prevalence of myopenia in SSc patients varies, with the reported prevalence ranging from 10.7 to 41.9%, depending on the diagnostic criteria and cut-off values used. The majority of SSc patients included in the studies were female, with percentages ranging from 84.4 to 92%. The average age of the patients ranged from 52 to 64 years [17, 32, 43–49].

Myopenia in SSc patients was associated with factors such as malnutrition [32, 43–45, 47, 48], low BMI [16, 45–47], lower fat mass [16, 45, 47], longer disease duration [43, 45, 47, 49], higher mRSS score [43, 44, 47, 48], decline in forced vital capacity [45], capillaroscopy patterns [16, 47] and reduced lung function (DLCO) [16, 45, 47].

Category	**Assessment**	**SSc specific assessment**
Find-cases	SARC-F questionnaire consisting of five items for self-reported information from patients regarding symptoms associated with sarcopenia, screening tool to assess the risk of sarcopenia in individuals in various healthcare settings, including community healthcare and clinical environments [33].	The combination of high diagnostic accuracy and feasibility makes SARC-F with the addition of age and body mass measurements (SARC-F + EBM) appropriate screening tool for routine care of patients with SSc. It can effectively identify individuals with the condition while being practical to use in everyday clinical practice [34].
Assess	Measurements of muscle strength. Low muscle strength could be measured as handgrip strength, as it has been shown to correspond well with strength in other areas of the body (cut-off value of <27 kg for men and < 16 kg women), or isometric torque methods can be used to measure lower limb strength [33]. A suitable measure is the chair stand test, which can be used as a proxy for the strength of the leg muscles (quadriceps) (cut-off value >15 s for five rises) [33].	In SSc patients with hand disability, lower limb strength can be measured using isometric torque or chair stand methods rather than handgrip strength [33].
Confirm	To confirm sarcopenia by detection of low muscle quantity and quality, DXA is advised in clinical practice, and DXA, BIA, CT or MRI in research studies (cut-off value appendicular skeletal muscle mass (ASM)/height2 < 7.0 kg/m^2 for men, and < 5.5 kg/m^2 for women) [33].	The skeletal muscle mass expressed as skeletal muscle area (SMA) and skeletal muscle index (SMI) at L1 level on chest CT was demonstrated to be an accurate measure that is useful for detecting myopenia in patients with SSc [35]. In SSc patients with skin involvement (fibrosis, digital ulcers), BIA is unlikely to be suitable for measuring muscle mass as it does not measure muscle mass directly but instead derives an estimate of muscle mass based on whole body electrical conductivity and may underestimate muscle mass in SSc patients [36].
Severity	Severity can be evaluated by performance measures; gait speed (≤0.8 m/s), short physical performance battery (SPPB) (≤8 points score), timed-up-and-go test (TUG) (≥20 s) and 400-m walk tests can be used (non-completion or ≥ 6 min for completion) [33].	

Table 1.
EWGSOP guidelines for diagnosis of sarcopenia recommend following the pathway: Find cases-assess-confirm-severity (F-A-C-S) [32].

Cachectic features are commonly observed in SSc patients with myopenia. The mechanisms underlying muscle wasting in SSc differ from those in other diseases and are primarily related to immunosuppression and malnutrition due to malabsorption syndrome [43]. As the disease progresses, the anabolic resistance caused by the vasculopathy may further accelerate the wasting of muscle and adipose tissue. Inflammation, neurological changes and polypharmacy may contribute to the progression from cachexia to sarcopenia in subsets of SSc patients.

Of the studies conducted with SSc patients, only two specifically address sarcopenia using the diagnostic criteria established by EWGSOP [32], or the AWGS criteria [44]. However, in several studies, the concept and definition of sarcopenia were not appropriate. The diagnosis was primarily based on individual assessment of skeletal muscle mass or muscle strength, without considering other factors contributing to sarcopenia, such as muscle quality [16, 45–47]. On the other hand, some studies focused on measuring body composition considering muscle mass or fat-free mass in SSc patients [43, 48, 49].

Studies that investigated sarcopenia in SSc patients showed prevalence between 22.5 and 22.7% [33, 37]. Potential predictors of sarcopenia in SSc patients were malnutrition, low body mass index (BMI), inflammation and number of immunosuppressants used. In addition, correlations between sarcopenia and disease subtype dSSc [46, 47] were observed. Sarcopenic SSc patients had a worse capillaroscopy pattern and lower quality of life as measured by the SF-36 survey [32, 47].

In summary, muscle impairment in SSc spans a spectrum ranging from myopenia to sarcopenia, with varying underlying mechanisms and severity. The interplay of immunosuppression, malnutrition, vasculopathy, inflammation and neurological alterations contributes to the muscle wasting and dysfunction observed in SSc patients. Further research is needed to better understand the specific mechanisms and the different subsets of muscle impairment in SSc patients.

4. Importance of non-myogenic cells in muscle pathology of SSs

In the histology of SSc muscles, interstitial and perivascular fibrosis are observed [6, 50]; however, the question remains, why is fibrosis in muscles not as frequent and as extensive as in skin.

Although myofibres are the major cell type in skeletal muscle, other cells are also important for the maintenance of muscle homeostasis. The essential components for the regeneration of muscle tissue are myogenic progenitor cells known as satellite cells. However, estimates in rats suggest that approximately half of all nuclei in skeletal muscles belong to non-muscle cells, including fibroblasts, endothelial cells and pericytes. Among these, fibroblasts are especially prominent [51]. They are associated with the formation of transient fibrosis that occurs following muscle injury, and, where repair is not successful, in the formation of resilient scar tissue, in addition to the gradual accumulation of muscle connective tissue that may occur with ageing (in sarcopenia) [52]. However, they are also implicated in regeneration, as 30 days after injury their number was increased fourfold and they were located preferentially surrounding regenerating muscle fibres. Even more, strong stimulation of myogenesis by fibroblasts was observed in cell culture, pointing towards direct stimulation of satellite cell differentiation and fusion [53]. More recent research found that these cells are fibro-adipogenic progenitors (FAP) that can differentiate into adipocytes or myofibroblasts and thus cause fibrosis and fatty infiltration, the two crucial processes of muscle degeneration and diseases (**Figure 5**) [55]. The fate of FAPs is strongly dependent on the microenvironment. Myokine IL-15 promotes skeletal muscle regeneration by stimulating the proliferation of FAPs and suppresses fatty infiltration by inhibiting their differentiation into adipocytes [54, 56]. In acute muscle injury, immune cells release IL-4 supporting FAP proliferation, while macrophages induce TNF-α-mediated FAP apoptosis shortly after entering the transient proregenerative phase [57]. Contrary, in chronic muscle injury, such as myositis, the macrophages switch from M1 to M2 and secrete TGF-β1, allowing FAPs to evade apoptosis and continue to secrete ECM components, resulting in fibrosis [57].

Some of the effects of FAP can be explained by the mediators that they secrete. FAPs are major producers of IL-6, IL-33 and follistatin after acute injury [54].

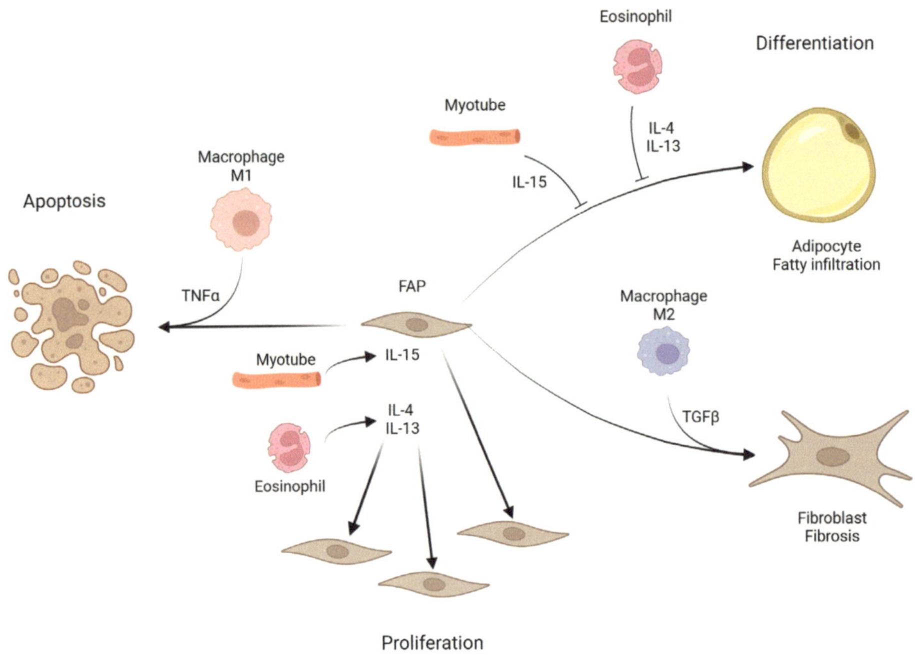

Figure 5.
Differentiation of fibro-adipogenic progenitors in skeletal muscle. Based on ref. [54].

5. Myokines

Skeletal muscle tissue is not only a component of the locomotor system but also a secretory organ, signalling through direct cell-cell interactions, cell surface molecules and soluble factors [58]. Contracting myofibres are a source of myokines, which exert their functions within the muscle tissue and in other organs such as adipose tissue, brain, liver, bone and pancreas [59]. Myokine signalling positively affects various biological processes, including metabolism, muscle hypertrophy and cognition, as well as tumour growth suppression and inflammation reduction [60]. Myokine molecules are also released from immune cells, possessing additional functions, often of an inflammatory nature, and can therefore also be classified as cytokines (**Figure 6**). However, further research is needed to identify the exact causes that could explain why, how and in what circumstances a molecule exerts its effects as a myokine or a cytokine.

Despite the positive effects, exercise is associated with acute inflammation, which is necessary for the repair of exercise-induced damage in the muscle tissue [61]. However, evidence indicates that physical exercise is safe and beneficial, as it does not exacerbate long-term inflammation or the number or degree of joint damage [59]. Long-term engagement in physical activity combined with reduced energy intake decreases the levels of systemic inflammatory markers, suggesting the downregulation of inflammation [59]. Moreover, it suppresses fibrotic processes and promotes circulation and vascular repair [62]. Caution is necessary for patients with interstitial lung disease who are at risk for oxygen desaturation during exercise [63].

The beneficial effects and safety of physical exercise make it an excellent non-pharmaceutical anti-inflammatory therapy for patients with SSc [59]. In SSc, muscle disuse often occurs because of difficulties with performing physical activities due

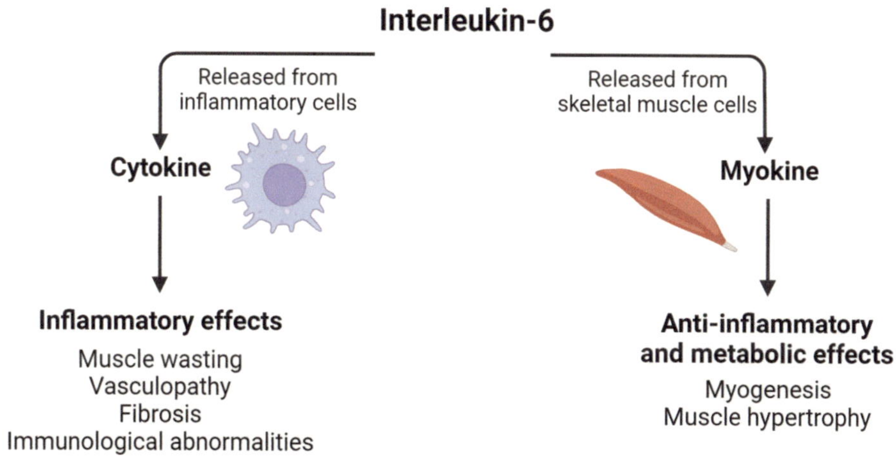

Figure 6.
Duality of IL-6 effects.

to common disease-related symptoms such as bone and muscle pain, stiffness and immobility. Muscle disuse exacerbates the symptoms, making it increasingly more difficult to break the cycle of physical inactivity [62]. Regular physical activity adjusted to the patient's abilities can relieve symptoms and improve physical health and psychosocial well-being. Physical activity interventions in patients with SSc have been reported to enhance general health parameters, including exercise tolerance, muscle strength and aerobic capacity, and provide symptom relief, as evidenced by improvement in handgrip strength, microstomia, pain and disability score [62].

5.1 IL-6

Among the factors that trigger IL-6 release from skeletal muscle cells are muscle contraction and reduced availability of metabolic substrates, which is why IL-6 is often referred to as the muscle energy sensor. IL-6 increases serum levels of cortisol, IL-1Ra (interleukin-1 receptor antagonist protein) and IL-10, which exert anti-inflammatory and metabolic effects [59]. As a myokine, IL-6 is essential for satellite cell-dependent myogenesis and overload-induced muscle hypertrophy (**Figure 6**) [64].

In contrast, when secreted in an inflammatory milieu or when its elevation and activity are prolonged, IL-6 is considered an inflammatory cytokine with the opposite effects on skeletal muscle, causing muscle wasting [65]. Elevated levels of IL-6 are associated with many inflammatory diseases, including SSc. Along with IL-4 and TGFβ, IL-6 is regarded as a fibrogenic cytokine, mediating its profibrotic actions by stimulating collagen production and inhibiting collagenase synthesis [26].

Consistent with its role in SSc-related inflammation and fibrosis, upregulation of IL-6 was shown in the following:

- Skin fibroblasts of SSc patients, where IL-6 levels correlate with the degree of collagen production [66],
- Serum of SSc patients, where IL-6 levels correlate with the disease severity [26, 66, 67],

- Exhaled breath and bronchoalveolar lavage of SSc patients, where IL-6 levels correlate with the extension of lung fibrosis [68].

The pathological role of IL-6 in SSc was demonstrated in experiments on animal SSc models, where IL-6 blockade or gene knockout resulted in the suppression of disease development [69].

IL-6 may have a role in all three features of the early stages of SSc pathogenesis: vasculopathy, immunological abnormalities and fibrosis [26]. *In vitro*, IL-6 can activate endothelial cells and induce their apoptosis leading to the development of endothelial damage [70]. Chronically elevated IL-6 leads to imbalances in cytokine levels and contributes to the proinflammatory and profibrotic phenotype in SSc [68]. IL-6 shifts the balance of naive T cell differentiation towards enhanced differentiation into Th17 and suppressed differentiation into Treg [66, 68]. This imbalance is associated with the loss of immunological tolerance, a characteristic of various autoimmune and inflammatory diseases [69]. Additionally, IL-6 directs the differentiation of T cells into Th2 cells, thus promoting the emergence of a Th2 phenotype, a typical cytokine profile observed in SSc [26]. Th2 cells secrete more IL-6, along with IL-4 and other Th2 cytokines, inducing a self-sustaining inflammatory loop [67]. This results in upregulated IL-6 synthesis in various cell types, namely B cells, PBMCs, T cells, NK cells, epithelial cells, alveolar monocytes and macrophages, and fibroblasts [26, 66–68].

In this regard, IL-6 seems to promote SSc pathogenesis; however, the contribution of the myokine portion or better lack of it, enables the dominance of negative effects and is not yet clear.

5.2 IL-15

Interleukin-15 is a proinflammatory cytokine crucial for the growth and survival of NK cells, B and T lymphocytes, eosinophils and mast cells. It is expressed in endothelial cells, vascular smooth muscle cells, fibroblasts, adipocytes, keratinocytes, cardiomyocytes and skeletal muscle cells [71]. There is a rapid increase in circulating levels of IL-15 in response to exercise. As a myokine, IL-15 regulates lipid metabolism and muscle regeneration. Skeletal muscle protects against excessive fat accumulation by releasing IL-15, which inhibits lipid deposition in preadipocytes and accumulation of visceral fat [59, 72].

In SSc, serum levels of IL-15 are elevated and correlate negatively with vital lung capacity, reflecting pulmonary fibrosis [71].

Its role in the transmigration and infiltration of immune cells may contribute to autoimmunity in SSc [71].

Although this correlation suggests a profibrotic effect of IL-15, results from *in vitro* experiments in healthy human lung foetal fibroblasts indicate that IL-15 reduces the extent of fibrosis by inhibiting TGFβ-mediated myofibroblast differentiation and type I collagen expression [73]. The interplay of IL-15 and TGFβ on SSc-derived fibroblasts remains to be elucidated, but in healthy fibroblasts, the upregulation of IL-15 may be a response to the increased activity of TGFβ to counteract its effects.

5.3 SPARC

Secreted Protein Acidic and Rich in Cysteine (SPARC), also known as osteonectin or basement-membrane protein 40 (BM-40), is a calcium-binding, extracellular matrix-associated glycoprotein released into the bloodstream by skeletal muscle in response to aerobic exercise. It mediates interactions between cells and their surrounding matrix by binding to ECM components, cellular receptors and secreted growth factors [74, 75]. It also induces the expression of proteases or their inhibitors and is thus important for the regulation of many processes involved in homeostasis and disease, such as cell proliferation, migration and invasion, tissue remodelling, angiogenesis, immune function, wound healing and fibrosis [74–76].

In SSc, SPARC appears to be involved in vasculopathy and fibrotic processes. By affecting cytoskeleton reorganisation and cell-ECM interactions, SPARC may induce intracellular gap formation in endothelial cells, leading to alterations in EC barrier function and increased paracellular permeability with perivascular oedema [77]. These are characteristics of SSc vasculopathy, along with the recruitment of inflammatory cells and intravascular platelet activation [78].

SPARC is commonly overexpressed in fibrotic tissue [79]. In SSc, SPARC overexpression was reported in dermal fibroblasts, endothelial cells, pericytes and epidermal keratinocytes [74]. The serum concentration of SPARC is elevated as well, but only in patients with limited SSc [75, 78]. The effects of SPARC on the development of a profibrotic phenotype seem to be associated with TGFβ, a driver of fibrotic processes [75, 79]. SPARC upregulates several ECM- and fibrosis-related genes in SSc dermal fibroblasts, contrary to dermal fibroblasts of healthy individuals, which do not respond to SPARC [75].

The difference between the responsiveness of healthy versus SSc-derived fibroblasts to SPARC is TGFβ-signalling dependent. TGFβ induces SPARC expression and vice versa, forming an autocrine feedback loop [80]. Additionally, SPARC enhances the cellular sensitivity to TGFβ by binding to the TGFβ receptor and altering its conformation, which results in increased expression of ECM- and fibrosis-related genes in cells exposed to both TGFβ and SPARC, compared to TGFβ only [81].

Accordingly, *in vitro* experiments showed the profibrotic effects of SPARC in SSc fibroblasts can be reversed by blocking the TGFβ receptor [75]. Furthermore, SPARC silencing results in decreased synthesis of collagen and connective tissue growth factor (CTGF) in fibroblasts obtained from SSc patients and alleviation of lung and skin fibrosis in bleomycin-induced fibrosis model [82–84].

5.4 LIF

Leukaemia Inhibitory Factor (LIF) is a myokine that acts by binding to its receptor LIFR and a signal transducer gp130, classifying LIF as a cytokine of the IL-6 family [85]. Its name derives from early research showing its ability to inhibit proliferation and induce differentiation of M1 myeloid leukaemia cells [86]. It is now known that LIF is highly pleiotropic, functioning in various processes across several organ systems such as haematopoiesis, embryogenesis, bone formation, skeletal and cardiac muscle and nervous system function [87]. In skeletal muscle, LIF is a contraction-induced myokine; however, no increases plasma levels were observed after exercise, pointing to local effects. LIFR is mainly expressed by satellite cells and LIF induces their proliferation and inhibits their premature differentiation [88]. Due to the angiostatic properties of LIF, loss of LIF function stimulates angiogenesis [89].

Serum levels of LIF are decreased in the early stages of SSc, as is the expression of LIF in SSc skin. Additionally, the expression of LIFR is downregulated in SSc skin in similar dynamics as LIF, while gp130 is downregulated irrespective of the disease stage [89]. Altered LIF function in the early stages of SSc might contribute to impaired angiostasis, leading to vasculopathy; however, it remains to be determined if LIF from muscles contributes to some potential effects in SSc or other tissues/cells contribute the majority.

6. Conclusions

Muscle involvement is a significant burden for patients with SSc and affects most of them. Clinically, muscle involvement is usually manifested by myalgia, muscle weakness and tenderness. Histologically, two main patterns can be identified in the skeletal muscles of SSc patients: fibrosing and inflammatory myopathy. The latter is associated with characteristic autoantibodies: anti-PM/Scl, anti-Ku, anti-U1RNP and anti-U3RNP. A large proportion of SSc patients with muscle involvement fulfil the criteria for both SSc and autoimmune myositis and can therefore be classified into a specific overlap SSc/AIM entity called scleromyositis.

Due to malnutrition, GIT involvement, inflammation, treatments and difficulty with engaging in physical exercise, SSc/AIM overlap patients often suffer from myopenia (muscle wasting), which can later develop into sarcopenia in approximately 20% of patients, which is associated with worse disease outcome and quality of life.

One aspect of muscle involvement in SSc is associated with changes in cellular function and the microenvironment in skeletal muscle tissue. However, essential cell types such as fibro-adipogenic progenitors and their role in SSc are incompletely understood. Their microenvironment depends largely on myokines secreted by contracting myotubes. Research on myokines suggests that some have beneficial and some deleterious effects on skeletal muscle in disease. Although some of the effects are well known, the challenge remains to accurately determine the amounts and effects of myokines released from muscle fibres as opposed to those released by other cell types.

Acknowledgements

This research was funded by the Slovenian Research Agency ARRS, with project J7-3153 and the National Research Program #P3-0314, P3-0043.

The figures were made with BioRender.

Conflict of interest

The authors declare no conflict of interest.

Appendices and nomenclature

AIM	autoimmune myositis
AWGS	Asian Working Group for Sarcopenia
BM-40	basement-membrane protein 40
BMI	body mass index
CK	creatinine kinase
CTGF	connective tissue growth factor
dcSSc	diffuse cutaneous systemic sclerosis
DLCO	diffusing capacity for carbon monoxid
ECM	extra-cellular matrix
EMG	electromyography
ENMC	European Neuro Muscular Centre
EUSTAR	European Scleroderma Trials and Research group

EWGSOP2	European Working Group on Sarcopenia in Older People
FAP	fibro-adipogenic progenitors
gp130	glycoprotein 130
IL-10	interleukin-10
IL-15	interleukin-15
IL-1Ra	interleukin-1 receptor antagonist protein
IL-4	interleukin-4
IL-6	interleukin-6
lcSSc	limited cutaneous systemic sclerosis
LIF	leukaemia inhibitory factor
LIFR	leukaemia inhibitory factor receptor
MHC-I	major histocompatibility complex class I
MRI	magnetic resonance imaging
mRSS	modified Rodnan skin score
NK	cells natural killer cells
NVC	nailfold videocapillaroscopy
PBMC	peripheral blood mononuclear cell
SF-36	36-item short form survey
SPARC	secreted protein acidic and rich in cysteine
SSc	systemic sclerosis
TGF-β1	transforming growth factor β
Th cells	T-helper cells
TNF-α	tumour necrosis factor α

Author details

Anja Srpčič[1,2], Felicita Urzi[3], Sanja Markez[1], Sergej Pirkmajer[2], Neža Brezovec[1], Katja Lakota[1,3] and Katja Perdan Pirkmajer[1,4]*

1 Department of Rheumatology, University Medical Centre Ljubljana, Slovenia

2 Institute of Pathophysiology, Faculty of Medicine, University of Ljubljana, Slovenia

3 FAMNIT, University of Primorska, Koper, Slovenia

4 Faculty of Medicine, Department of Internal Medicine, University of Ljubljana, Slovenia

*Address all correspondence to: katja.perdanpirkmajer@kclj.si

References

[1] Moinzadeh P, Kuhr K, Siegert E, Mueller-Ladner U, Riemekasten G, Gunther C, et al. Older age onset of systemic sclerosis - accelerated disease progression in all disease subsets. Rheumatology (Oxford, England). 2020;**59**(11):3380-3389

[2] Peoples C, Medsger TA Jr, Lucas M, Rosario BL, Feghali-Bostwick CA. Gender differences in systemic sclerosis: Relationship to clinical features, serologic status and outcomes. Journal of Scleroderma and Related Disorders. 2016;**1**(2):177-240

[3] Hughes M, Herrick AL. Systemic sclerosis. British Journal of Hospital Medicine (London, England). 2019;**80**(9):530-536

[4] Lorand V, Czirjak L, Minier T. Musculoskeletal involvement in systemic sclerosis. Presse Médicale. 2014;**43**(10 Pt. 2):e315-e328

[5] Martin Calderon L, Chaudhary M, Pope JE. Healthcare utilization and economic burden in systemic sclerosis: A systematic review. Rheumatology (Oxford, England). 2022;**61**(8):3123-3131

[6] Walker UA, Clements PJ, Allanore Y, Distler O, Oddis CV, Khanna D, et al. Muscle involvement in systemic sclerosis: Points to consider in clinical trials. Rheumatology (Oxford, England). 2017;**56**(Suppl. 5):v38-v44

[7] Zhou M, Jiang L, Nie L, Chen T, Zhang T, Sun W, et al. Myopathy is a risk factor for poor prognosis of patients with systemic sclerosis: A retrospective cohort study. Medicine (Baltimore). 2020;**99**(33):e21734

[8] Giannini M, Ellezam B, Leclair V, Lefebvre F, Troyanov Y, Hudson M, et al. Scleromyositis: A distinct novel entity within the systemic sclerosis and autoimmune myositis spectrum. Implications for care and pathogenesis. Frontiers in Immunology. 2022;**13**:974078

[9] Jung M, Bonner A, Hudson M, Baron M, Pope JE, Canadian Scleroderma Research G. Myopathy is a poor prognostic feature in systemic sclerosis: Results from the Canadian scleroderma research group (CSRG) cohort. Scandinavian Journal of Rheumatology. 2014;**43**(3):217-220

[10] Bratoiu I, Burlui AM, Cardoneanu A, Macovei LA, Richter P, Rusu-Zota G, et al. The involvement of smooth muscle, striated muscle, and the myocardium in scleroderma: A review. International Journal of Molecular Sciences. 2022;**23**(19):12011

[11] Paik JJ, Wigley FM, Mejia AF, Hummers LK. Independent association of severity of muscle weakness with disability as measured by the health assessment questionnaire disability index in scleroderma. Arthritis Care & Research (Hoboken). 2016;**68**(11):1695-1703

[12] Walker UA, Tyndall A, Czirjak L, Denton C, Farge-Bancel D, Kowal-Bielecka O, et al. Clinical risk assessment of organ manifestations in systemic sclerosis: A report from the EULAR scleroderma trials and research group database. Annals of the Rheumatic Diseases. 2007;**66**(6):754-763

[13] Meyer OC, Fertig N, Lucas M, Somogyi N, Medsger TA. Disease subsets, antinuclear antibody profile, and clinical features in 127 French and 247 US adult patients with systemic sclerosis. The Journal of Rheumatology. 2007;**34**(1):104-109

[14] Paik JJ, Wigley FM, Lloyd TE, Corse AM, Casciola-Rosen L, Shah AA, et al. Spectrum of muscle histopathologic findings in forty-two scleroderma patients with weakness. Arthritis Care & Research (Hoboken). 2015;**67**(10):1416-1425

[15] Corallo C, Cutolo M, Volpi N, Franci D, Agliano M, Montella A, et al. Histopathological findings in systemic sclerosis-related myopathy: Fibrosis and microangiopathy with lack of cellular inflammation. Therapeutic Advances in Musculoskeletal Disease. 2017;**9**(1):3-10

[16] Paolino SGF, Cimmino MA, Casabella A, Pizzorni C, Patanè M, Schenone C, et al. Advanced microvascular damage associated with occurence of sarcopenia in systemic sclerosis patients: Results from a retrospective cohort study. Clinical and Experimental Rheumatology. 2020;**38**:65-72

[17] Paolino S, Gotelli E, Goegan F, Casabella A, Ferrari G, Patane M, et al. Body composition and bone status in relation to microvascular damage in systemic sclerosis patients. Journal of Endocrinological Investigation. 2021;**44**(2):255-264

[18] Dumitru RB, Goodall AF, Broadbent DA, Del Galdo F, Tan AL, Biglands JD, et al. First pilot study of extracellular volume MRI measurement in peripheral muscle of systemic sclerosis patients suggests diffuse fibrosis. Rheumatology (Oxford, England). 2022;**61**(4):1651-1657

[19] Selva-O'Callaghan A, Guillen-Del-Castillo A, Gil-Vila A, Trallero-Araguás E, Matas-García A, Milisenda JC, et al. Systemic sclerosis-associated myopathy: How to treat. Current Treatment Options in Rheumatology. 2023. pp. 1-17

[20] Paik JJ, Wigley FM, Shah AA, Corse AM, Casciola-Rosen L, Hummers LK, et al. Association of Fibrosing Myopathy in systemic sclerosis and higher mortality. Arthritis Care & Research (Hoboken). 2017;**69**(11):1764-1770

[21] Leclair V, D'Aoust J, Gyger G, Landon-Cardinal O, Meyer A, O'Ferrall E, et al. Autoantibody profiles delineate distinct subsets of scleromyositis. Rheumatology (Oxford, England). 2022;**61**(3):1148-1157

[22] Junior JG, Mugii N, Inaoka PT, Sampaio-Barros PD, Shinjo SK. Inflammatory myopathies overlapping with systemic sclerosis: A systematic review. Clinical Rheumatology. 2022;**41**(7):1951-1963

[23] Bhansing KJ, van Riel PL, van Engelen BG, Fransen J, Vonk MC. Patients with systemic sclerosis/polymyositis overlap have a worse survival rate than patients without it. The Journal of Rheumatology. 2016;**43**(10):1838-1843

[24] Bhansing KJ, Lammens M, Knaapen HK, van Riel PL, van Engelen BG, Vonk MC. Scleroderma-polymyositis overlap syndrome versus idiopathic polymyositis and systemic sclerosis: A descriptive study on clinical features and myopathology. Arthritis Research & Therapy. 2014;**16**(3):R111

[25] Lefebvre F, Giannini M, Ellezam B, Leclair V, Troyanov Y, Hoa S, et al. Histopathological features of systemic sclerosis-associated myopathy: A scoping review. Autoimmunity Reviews. 2021;**20**(7):102851

[26] Brown M, O'Reilly S. The immunopathogenesis of fibrosis in systemic sclerosis. Clinical

and Experimental Immunology. 2019;**195**(3):310-321

[27] Fearon K, Evans WJ, Anker SD. Myopenia-a new universal term for muscle wasting. Journal of Cachexia, Sarcopenia and Muscle. 2011;**2**(1):1-3

[28] Evans WJ, Morley JE, Argiles J, Bales C, Baracos V, Guttridge D, et al. Cachexia: A new definition. Clinical Nutrition. 2008;**27**(6):793-799

[29] Berardi E, Madaro L, Lozanoska-Ochser B, Adamo S, Thorrez L, Bouche M, et al. A pound of flesh: What cachexia is and what it is not. Diagnostics (Basel). 2021;**11**(1):116

[30] Anker SD, Morley JE, von Haehling S. Welcome to the ICD-10 code for sarcopenia. Journal of Cachexia, Sarcopenia and Muscle. 2016;7(5):512-514

[31] Rosenberg IH. Sarcopenia: Origins and clinical relevance. The Journal of Nutrition. 1997;**127**(Suppl. 5):990S-991S

[32] Siegert E, March C, Otten L, Makowka A, Preis E, Buttgereit F, et al. Prevalence of sarcopenia in systemic sclerosis: Assessing body composition and functional disability in patients with systemic sclerosis. Nutrition. 2018;**55-56**:51-55

[33] Cruz-Jentoft AJ, Bahat G, Bauer J, Boirie Y, Bruyere O, Cederholm T, et al. Sarcopenia: Revised European consensus on definition and diagnosis. Age and Ageing. 2019;**48**(1):16-31

[34] Hax V, do Espirito Santo RC, Dos Santos LP, Farinon M, de Oliveira MS, Tres GL, et al. Practical screening tools for sarcopenia in patients with systemic sclerosis. PLoS One. 2021;**16**(1):e0245683

[35] da Rocha DS, Tessari JA, Mainardi NB, Hax V, Gasparin AA, de Oliveira CAV, et al. Assessment of muscle mass using chest computed tomography-based quantitative and qualitative measurements in patients with systemic sclerosis: A retrospective study with cross-sectional and longitudinal analyses. Seminars in Arthritis and Rheumatism. 2023;**59**:152168

[36] Kyle UG, Bosaeus I, De Lorenzo AD, Deurenberg P, Elia M, Manuel Gomez J, et al. Bioelectrical impedance analysis-part II: Utilization in clinical practice. Clinical Nutrition. 2004;**23**(6):1430-1453

[37] Bauer JM. Muscle function and sarcopenia: Clinical implications of recent research. Journal of the American Medical Directors Association. 2021;**22**(4):725-727

[38] Narici M, McPhee J, Conte M, Franchi MV, Mitchell K, Tagliaferri S, et al. Age-related alterations in muscle architecture are a signature of sarcopenia: The ultrasound sarcopenia index. Journal of Cachexia, Sarcopenia and Muscle. 2021;**12**(4):973-982

[39] Fragala MS, Fukuda DH, Stout JR, Townsend JR, Emerson NS, Boone CH, et al. Muscle quality index improves with resistance exercise training in older adults. Experimental Gerontology. 2014;**53**:1-6

[40] Ferri E, Marzetti E, Calvani R, Picca A, Cesari M, Arosio B. Role of age-related mitochondrial dysfunction in sarcopenia. International Journal of Molecular Sciences. 2020;**21**(15):5236

[41] Hepple RT. When motor unit expansion in ageing muscle fails, atrophy ensues. The Journal of Physiology. 2018;**596**(9):1545-1546

[42] Li CW, Yu K, Shyh-Chang N, Jiang Z, Liu T, Ma S, et al. Pathogenesis

of sarcopenia and the relationship with fat mass: Descriptive review. Journal of Cachexia, Sarcopenia and Muscle. 2022;**13**(2):781-794

[43] Rosato E, Gigante A, Pellicano C, Villa A, Iannazzo F, Alunni Fegatelli D, et al. Symptoms related to gastrointestinal tract involvement and low muscularity in systemic sclerosis. Clinical Rheumatology. 2022;**41**(6):1687-1696

[44] Sangaroon A, Foocharoen C, Theerakulpisut D, Srichompoo K, Mahakkanukrauh A, Suwannaroj S, et al. Prevalence and clinical association of sarcopenia among Thai patients with systemic sclerosis. Scientific Reports. 2022;**12**(1):18198

[45] Caimmi C, Caramaschi P, Venturini A, Bertoldo E, Vantaggiato E, Viapiana O, et al. Malnutrition and sarcopenia in a large cohort of patients with systemic sclerosis. Clinical Rheumatology. 2018;**37**(4):987-997

[46] Allen TS, Southwood CR, Doerfler BM, Hirano I, Sheean PM. The impact of medical nutrition therapy for patients with advanced systemic sclerosis (MNT PASS). Journal of the Academy of Nutrition and Dietetics. 2014;**114**(9):A44

[47] Corallo C, Fioravanti A, Tenti S, Pecetti G, Nuti R, Giordano N. Sarcopenia in systemic sclerosis: The impact of nutritional, clinical, and laboratory features. Rheumatology International. 2019;**39**(10):1767-1775

[48] Sari A, Esme M, Aycicek GS, Armagan B, Kilic L, Ertenli AI, et al. Evaluating skeletal muscle mass with ultrasound in patients with systemic sclerosis. Nutrition. 2021;**84**:110999

[49] Marighela TF, Genaro PS, Pinheiro MM, Szejnfeld VL, Kayser C. Risk factors for body composition abnormalities in systemic sclerosis. Clinical Rheumatology. 2013;**32**(7):1037-1044

[50] Medsger TA Jr, Rodnan GP, Moossy J, Vester JW. Skeletal muscle involvement in progressive systemic sclerosis (scleroderma). Arthritis and Rheumatism. 1968;**11**(4):554-568

[51] Schmalbruch H, Hellhammer U. The number of nuclei in adult rat muscles with special reference to satellite cells. The Anatomical Record. 1977;**189**(2):169-175

[52] Mendias CL. Fibroblasts take the Centre stage in human skeletal muscle regeneration. The Journal of Physiology. 2017;**595**(15):5005

[53] Mackey AL, Magnan M, Chazaud B, Kjaer M. Human skeletal muscle fibroblasts stimulate in vitro myogenesis and in vivo muscle regeneration. The Journal of Physiology. 2017;**595**(15):5115-5127

[54] Biferali B, Proietti D, Mozzetta C, Madaro L. Fibro-Adipogenic progenitors cross-talk in skeletal muscle: The social network. Frontiers in Physiology. 2019;**10**:1074

[55] Kang X, Yang MY, Shi YX, Xie MM, Zhu M, Zheng XL, et al. Interleukin-15 facilitates muscle regeneration through modulation of fibro/adipogenic progenitors. Cell Communication and Signaling: CCS. 2018;**16**(1):42

[56] Chen W, You W, Valencak TG, Shan T. Bidirectional roles of skeletal muscle fibro-adipogenic progenitors in homeostasis and disease. Ageing Research Reviews. 2022;**80**:101682

[57] Lemos DR, Babaeijandaghi F, Low M, Chang CK, Lee ST, Fiore D,

et al. Nilotinib reduces muscle fibrosis in chronic muscle injury by promoting TNF-mediated apoptosis of fibro/adipogenic progenitors. Nature Medicine. 2015;**21**(7):786-794

[58] Nelke C, Dziewas R, Minnerup J, Meuth SG, Ruck T. Skeletal muscle as potential central link between sarcopenia and immune senescence. eBioMedicine. 2019;**49**:381-388

[59] Benatti FB, Pedersen BK. Exercise as an anti-inflammatory therapy for rheumatic diseases-myokine regulation. Nature Reviews Rheumatology. 2015;**11**(2):86-97

[60] Severinsen MCK, Pedersen BK. Muscle-organ crosstalk: The emerging roles of Myokines. Endocrine Reviews. 2020;**41**(4):594-609

[61] Cerqueira E, Marinho DA, Neiva HP, Lourenco O. Inflammatory effects of high and moderate intensity exercise-a systematic review. Frontiers in Physiology. 2019;**10**:1550

[62] Pettersson H, Alexanderson H, Poole JL, Varga J, Regardt M, Russell AM, et al. Exercise as a multi-modal disease-modifying medicine in systemic sclerosis: An introduction by the global fellowship on rehabilitation and exercise in systemic sclerosis (G-FoRSS). Best Practice & Research. Clinical Rheumatology. 2021;**35**(3):101695

[63] Someya F, Mugii N, Hasegawa M, Yahata T, Nakagawa T. Predictors of exercise-induced oxygen desaturation in systemic sclerosis patients with interstitial lung disease. Respiratory Care. 2014;**59**(1):75-80

[64] Munoz-Canoves P, Scheele C, Pedersen BK, Serrano AL. Interleukin-6 myokine signaling in skeletal muscle: A double-edged sword? The FEBS Journal. 2013;**280**(17):4131-4148

[65] Moresi V, Adamo S, Berghella L. The JAK/STAT pathway in skeletal muscle pathophysiology. Frontiers in Physiology. 2019;**10**:500

[66] Muangchan C, Pope JE. Interleukin 6 in systemic sclerosis and potential implications for targeted therapy. The Journal of Rheumatology. 2012;**39**(6):1120-1124

[67] Muangchant C, Pope JE. The significance of interleukin-6 and C-reactive protein in systemic sclerosis: A systematic literature review. Clinical and Experimental Rheumatology. 2013;**31**(2 Suppl. 76):122-134

[68] Baraut J, Michel L, Verrecchia F, Farge D. Relationship between cytokine profiles and clinical outcomes in patients with systemic sclerosis. Autoimmunity Reviews. 2010;**10**(2):65-73

[69] Tanaka T, Narazaki M, Kishimoto T. IL-6 in inflammation, immunity, and disease. Cold Spring Harbor Perspectives in Biology. 2014;**6**(10):a016295

[70] Barnes TC, Spiller DG, Anderson ME, Edwards SW, Moots RJ. Endothelial activation and apoptosis mediated by neutrophil-dependent interleukin 6 trans-signalling: A novel target for systemic sclerosis? Annals of the Rheumatic Diseases. 2011;**70**(2):366-372

[71] Wuttge DM, Wildt M, Geborek P, Wollheim FA, Scheja A, Akesson A. Serum IL-15 in patients with early systemic sclerosis: A potential novel marker of lung disease. Arthritis Research & Therapy. 2007;**9**(5):R85

[72] Nadeau L, Aguer C. Interleukin-15 as a myokine: Mechanistic insight into

its effect on skeletal muscle metabolism. Applied Physiology, Nutrition, and Metabolism. 2019;**44**(3):229-238

[73] Wuttge DM, Wildt M, Scheja A, Westergren-Thorsson G. Interleukin-15 attenuates transforming growth factor-beta1-induced myofibroblast differentiation in human fetal lung fibroblasts. European Cytokine Network. 2010;**21**(3):165-176

[74] Davies CA, Jeziorska M, Freemont AJ, Herrick AL. Expression of osteonectin and matrix Gla protein in scleroderma patients with and without calcinosis. Rheumatology (Oxford, England). 2006;**45**(11):1349-1355

[75] Carvalheiro T, Malvar Fernandez B, Ottria A, Giovannone B, Marut W, Reedquist KA, et al. Extracellular SPARC cooperates with TGF-beta signalling to induce pro-fibrotic activation of systemic sclerosis patient dermal fibroblasts. Rheumatology (Oxford, England). 2020;**59**(9):2258-2263

[76] Zhou X, Tan FK, Reveille JD, Wallis D, Milewicz DM, Ahn C, et al. Association of novel polymorphisms with the expression of SPARC in normal fibroblasts and with susceptibility to scleroderma. Arthritis and Rheumatism. 2002;**46**(11):2990-2999

[77] Young BA, Wang P, Goldblum SE. The counteradhesive protein SPARC regulates an endothelial paracellular pathway through protein tyrosine phosphorylation. Biochemical and Biophysical Research Communications. 1998;**251**(1):320-327

[78] Macko RFGA, Young BA, Lowitt MH, White B, Wigley FM, Goldblum SE. Increased circulating concentrations of the counteradhesive proteins SPARC and thrombospondin-1 in systemic sclerosis (scleroderma). Relationship to platelet and endothelial cell activation. The Journal of Rheumatology. 2002;**29**(12):2565-2570

[79] Ding W, Pu W, Jiang S, Ma Y, Liu Q, Wu W, et al. Evaluation of the antifibrotic potency by knocking down SPARC, CCR2 and SMAD3. eBioMedicine. 2018;**38**:238-247

[80] Scavelli K, Chatterjee A, Rhee DJ. Secreted protein acidic and rich in cysteine in ocular tissue. Journal of Ocular Pharmacology and Therapeutics. 2015;**31**(7):396-405

[81] Francki A, McClure TD, Brekken RA, Motamed K, Murri C, Wang T, et al. SPARC regulates TGF-beta1-dependent signaling in primary glomerular mesangial cells. Journal of Cellular Biochemistry. 2004;**91**(5):915-925

[82] Zhou X, Tan FK, Guo X, Arnett FC. Attenuation of collagen production with small interfering RNA of SPARC in cultured fibroblasts from the skin of patients with scleroderma. Arthritis and Rheumatism. 2006;**54**(8):2626-2631

[83] Strandjord TP, Madtes DK, Weiss DJ, Sage EH. Collagen accumulation is decreased in SPARC-null mice with bleomycin-induced pulmonary fibrosis. The American Journal of Physiology. 1999;**277**(3):L628-L635

[84] Wang JC, Lai S, Guo X, Zhang X, de Crombrugghe B, Sonnylal S, et al. Attenuation of fibrosis in vitro and in vivo with SPARC siRNA. Arthritis Research & Therapy. 2010;**12**(2):R60

[85] Jorgensen MM, de la Puente P. Leukemia inhibitory factor: An important cytokine in pathologies and cancer. Biomolecules. 2022;**12**(2):217

[86] Gearing DP, Gough NM, King JA, Hilton DJ, Nicola NA, Simpson RJ,

et al. Molecular cloning and expression of cDNA encoding a murine myeloid leukaemia inhibitory factor (LIF). The EMBO Journal. 1987;**6**(13):3995-4002

[87] Metcalf D. The unsolved enigmas of leukemia inhibitory factor. Stem Cells. 2003;**21**(1):5-14

[88] Broholm C, Pedersen BK. Leukaemia inhibitory factor–An exercise-induced myokine. Exercise Immunology Review. 2010;**16**:77-85

[89] Taniguchi T, Miyagawa T, Tamaki Z, Nakamura K, Yamashita T, Saigusa R, et al. A possible implication of reduced levels of LIF, LIFR, and gp130 in vasculopathy related to systemic sclerosis. Archives of Dermatological Research. 2017;**309**(10):833-842